Death by Sitting

by DR. ERIC SOEHNGEN

DEDICATION

To my patients, with whom I have had the honour of consulting, and who suffer daily from the various effects of 'sitting disease.' Each of you has taught me more than medical school ever could. This book is for you.

And, perhaps most of all, I dedicate this book to the next generation. You have the ability to reshape our schools, universities, offices and cities. I will continue to support you in that effort.

CONTENTS

PREFACE

When it comes to furthering our understanding of human physiology and disease, it is one of the most exciting times in human history to be alive. Our bodies are the most fascinating and complex machines, and modern science has continued to unveil the full potential we carry within each of us. Through ongoing exploration of the body's fundamental interconnectivity of physical, mental and emotional elements – and with the support of state-of-the-art medical tools available today – we can seek to enhance human longevity and wellbeing. This has become not only the focus of my professional career, but my life's passion.

Over the years, I have been involved in numerous therapeutic studies where, due to extraordinary circumstances leading to ethical considerations, research would need to be prematurely halted. There were instances where one of the drugs, treatments or methods being measured proved to be significantly more effective than the other, so much so that it would be morally reprehensible to see the study to completion, whereby not allowing one group of probands (individuals involved in the study) to benefit from the undeniably superior treatment.

Dear reader, we find ourselves in the middle of the same scenario today, with just one key difference: that the study is taking place in the real world and each of us are participants. The key metric being studied is sitting vs. not sitting.

A generation ago, the world faced quite a similar situation with smoking tobacco. The evidence, that cigarette smoking is linked to numerous severe health issues, rapidly mounted study after study. Nevertheless, it took decades until we gained a significant level of public awareness regarding the associated risks; today, the danger of smoking is largely considered an undeniable truth and basic knowledge. If the human race were to improve in one regard as a whole, it should be to learn from those who came before us and to avoid repeating the same mistakes.

The Italian polymath Galileo Galilei (1564-1642) is famous for his standpoint that science has the responsibility – if not the obligation – to inform the public about groundbreaking discoveries, despite any and all opposition.

Fast forward half a century, and once again we find that it is time to reveal highly concerning scientific observations that must reshape how we live and work every day. The need for movement is so deeply ingrained within our innate composition – our hunter-gatherer genome – that we simply cannot ignore it. By continuing to turn a blind eye, when we often sit for more than eight hours each day, humans will inevitably pay an unnecessary death toll and ultimately lose the battle against the chronic 'societal-based diseases,' both as individuals as well as on a larger socioeconomic scale.

My professional journey through the universe of medical institutions and research laboratories has granted me personal insight into the fates of thousands of patients across cultures and continents. It is no exaggeration to say that I have seen great suffering, which in many cases was highly preventable. Oftentimes, the affected weren't even aware of how their daily actions could result in such unbearable chronic pain.

From my scientific findings, I came to the unwavering conclusion that I needed to change my position on this battlefield if I were to make a meaningful difference. Remaining in medicine and research would mean that I would continue to treat and investigate the *symptoms* of a disease, rather than working on a *treatment* or, even better, a method for *prevention*.

So, in 2016 I turned my full attention and effort towards developing a true alternative to the chair. I found a comrade in the office furniture industry who was equally enthusiastic about the challenge at hand. Together we founded Walkolution. Our company has been built on a core mission: to reimagine the modern office where our human genetic needs are at the very centre. At the same time, Walkolution seeks to foster and actively support this change for generations to come, starting with our school systems.

I believe that people in the second half of the 21st century will look back on our current sedentary lifestyle era with disbelief and shaking heads.

We can no longer take this sitting down. It is time for a movement revolution. This book will explain why.

Eric Soehngen, MD

INTRODUCTION

I am a huge believer in the proverbial 'elevator pitch.' In cases where important concepts or ideas may be considered too complex to be understood or appreciated by those unfamiliar with the subject matter, it is essential that one is able to boil the message down to just the essentials.

So what is the message of this book in just two sentences?

The human body's genetic imprint clearly indicates that we were designed to be active throughout the majority of the day. If, during our waking hours, we instead remain seated for six or more hours daily, we will inevitably ruin our physical and mental health and dramatically reduce our life expectancy.

Still a long way to go

It's natural to wonder how modern society could have missed such an important point up to now. Why have we just started to learn about the health risks associated with sedentariness in the last decade or so?

Part of the explanation is that it takes considerable time for the outcome of research studies to spread. In medical or epidemiological research settings, results are typically first shared amongst the scientific community within conferences and scientific publications. Only a fraction of studies ever reach any public awareness. Scientific parlance and the sheer complexity of most published studies also make it challenging or even impossible for the general public or press to follow up.

You are likely familiar with the mantra, "Sitting is the new smoking." Dr. James Levine, one of the pioneers in the research of the modern 'sitting disease,' was a driving force in bringing awareness to the larger public. His memorable statement has made headlines all over the world and triggered a greater awareness and interest in the topic.

Sitting has been widely overlooked as an independent risk factor for its long-term contribution to chronic diseases. However, with continually mounting evidence, the predominant opinion in the scientific and medical community has begun to change dramatically; we can now definitively say that a sedentary lifestyle contributes to heart disease, diabetes, cancer, dementia, and many other severe diseases. With the recommendation to reduce sitting time now appearing in official clinical guidelines, we can see that awareness is finally spreading beyond industry publications and is beginning to reach the 'real world.'

Despite numerous public and corporate campaigns to incorporate more movement in schools, universities and workplaces, sitting for eight to ten hours a day is still the global average. Reducing that duration to a safe amount is easier said than done, particularly since the social and professional context often leaves us no other choice but to sit. Students in the university library or lecture hall, office workers behind their desks or in meetings, people on their daily commute all face the same dilemma. It all adds up without us noticing and, in addition to all that, we spend even more time sitting during leisure time, for meals and in front of screens of all sizes.

How does sitting affect the body?

Upper back, neck and shoulders

The typical position at a desk, with the neck and head bent forward while working at a computer, leads to a host of spinal problems, chronic strains, headaches and herniated discs.

Lower back

Sitting puts enormous pressure on the spine, mostly at critical junctions in the lumbar spine and lower back, resulting in herniated discs, chronic back pain and spinal degeneration. Many also suffer mental effects from back pain, all too often leading to overprescription and opioid abuse.

Hips and glutes

Lack of extension in the hip muscles lead to tightness and a reduced range of motion, while weakened glute muscles decrease a person's stability. Both of these effects can lead to an increased risk for falls, particularly within the elderly population. Furthermore, nerve compression can lead to chronic repetitive radiating pain throughout the legs.

Abdominal muscles

Chronically weakened abdominal muscles further contribute to spinal problems due to lack of counterbalance, increasing the risk for long-term spinal damage, herniated discs and chronic back pain.

Bones

Chronic lack of movement leads to decreased bone density, paving the way towards osteoporosis, and an increased risk of fractures.

Lungs

While sitting at a desk, with hunched shoulders and a rounded spine, we experience a substantial reduction in our lung capacity, which is exacerbated by a lack of diaphragmatic movement due to abdominal compression between the upper body and the flexed hip. Over time, breathing becomes chronically impaired, leading to decreased energy and negative effects on the brain, including impaired focus and reduced memory.

Pancreas and metabolism

The body's ability to effectively respond to sugar intake is profoundly affected by prolonged sitting, leading to insulin resistance and diabetes. Long-term increased blood sugar levels give rise to cardiovascular disease, stroke, kidney failure, nerve damage, blindness and limb amputations, all of which can seriously lower the quality and expectancy of one's life.

Heart and blood vessels

Sitting leads to overall slower blood flow and a weakened heart muscle, resulting in higher blood pressure and chronic inflammation in the blood vessels. The combination of unhealthy accumulation of body fat and reduced muscle mass leads to higher unhealthy fats circulating in the blood, resulting in an increased risk for heart attack and stroke. Sitting for more than seven hours each day means an 85% increased risk of death from cardiovascular disease.

For every two hours a person spends sitting each day, the risk for cardiovascular disease increases by an additional 5%. Sitting also increases the levels of stress hormones and impairs blood circulation in the legs, which can damage leg veins (varicosis) and lead to the development of blood clots known as deep vein thrombosis.

Overweight

Sitting too long influences the dopamine and leptin hormones, which play an important role in the regulation of hunger and satiety. Weight gain as a result of inactivity can start a vicious cycle, in which it becomes harder and harder for people to lose weight.

Being overweight or obese increases the risk of a number of serious conditions, including diabetes, hypertension, heart disease and heart attack, stroke, cancer, kidney disease and liver disease; it can also result in sleep disturbances and cause a range of musculoskeletal problems.

Cancer

Sitting increases the risk for lung cancer by 54%, uterine cancer by 66% and colon cancer by 30%. This is likely due to hormonal changes (IGF-1), excessive insulin secretion, a state of constant inflammation and decreased production of antioxidant enzymes.

Obesity has also been linked to cancers involving the esophagus (gullet), stomach, liver, blood, brain, pancreas, colon (intestine), gallbladder, breasts and ovaries.

Digestion and bowels

Sitting after a meal causes food to compress in the intestines, which impairs digestion and can lead to long-term low level inflammation in and around the intestine with negative effects on the healthy gut flora (microbiome). This has been associated with diseases affecting the bowels, and can also contribute to allergies, asthma, metabolic syndrome, heart disease and cancer.

Brain

Movement triggers the release of neurochemicals, which are essential for awareness, proper memory function and mood stability.

The brain functions like a muscle. Without enough movement, the brain virtually shrinks in size, increasing the risk of developing depression, anxiety, dementia (including Alzheimer's disease), attention deficit disorder and more. An impaired response to stress can negatively impact numerous other organs, including the heart through the vegetative nervous system and the gut microflora / the microbiome with further implications for our cognitive and psychological wellbeing.

Exercise and standing cannot reverse the effects of sitting

Studies overwhelmingly show that even intense daily exercise can simply not undo the health risks that result from sitting for the majority of our waking hours. While exercise is certainly good for us and comes with countless health benefits, prolonged sedentary time is independently associated with the aforementioned risks, regardless of the amount of time an individual spends engaged in physical activity.

To explain why exercise alone is not enough, we have to look at what happens in the sedentary body. When we sit, the muscles in the legs don't contract and therefore don't pump blood back through the body – most importantly to the brain – and instead pool in the legs. Over time, this means that our large leg muscles require less fuel, decreasing our energy expenditure. The brain has a high, steady demand for energy in the form of glucose. A lack of glucose supply is interpreted by the brain as some kind of starvation risk, which triggers the release of hormones and gene regulation in a way that rapidly increases the level of blood sugar and decreases the level of fat burning. This response makes sense as a physiological survival mechanism. In today's world, however, when triggered by prolonged daily sitting time, this can soon turn into a major health risk, regardless of whether the person is an athlete who exercises regularly.

As a consequence, exercise time and sedentary time are two completely different entities, which need to be addressed separately. While we should try to engage in vigorous physically exercise for about 30-45 minutes a day, we should also ensure that time spent sitting doesn't add up to more than four hours on a daily basis.

A movement revolution is needed

More and more scientific evidence directly links inactivity and sedentariness to some of the most pressing health risks of our times. Effective countermeasures that provide a realistic outlook on preventing or reversing the effects of this 'sitting disease' are urgently needed, particularly as we consider the exploding healthcare costs associated with the treatment of chronically ill patients and the associated loss of productivity. At the same time, we are moving towards a society in which personal health and mental wellbeing have a higher meaning than ever before. We have the opportunity to witness and contribute to the changing landscape of companies and cities that have an ever increasing awareness for innovative health programs and which are beginning to see movement as a basic human right and need. We are just now taking the first steps towards transformation.

CHAPTER ONE:
HOW SITTING AFFECTS
THE MUSCULOSKELETAL SYSTEM

BIOMECHANICAL EVOLUTION

The human body has evolved to become a phenomenal machine capable of previously unfathomable feats. Athletes, such as Usain Bolt from Jamaica, have run 100 metres in just 9.58 seconds, with a top speed clocked at 27.8 mph. Others can jump higher than they stand tall, including world record holder Javier Sotomayor, who jumped 2.45 metres in the 1993 Olympic high jump competition representing Cuba. And, while these days many struggle to carry their groceries home, in 1985, American weightlifter Paul Edward Anderson hoisted an incredible 6,270 pounds in a back lift – the greatest weight ever lifted by a human.

Evolution has made humans the ultimate super-predator, able to move quickly and efficiently to hunt and gather food, and to even track prey over hundreds of kilometres as persistence hunters. In fact, this was our primary role and function for the vast majority of our time as humans on this planet. It is only in recent history that physical effort and stamina have become pursuits of personal interest or leisure.

Today, humans continue to show great interest and respect for these fantastic displays of stamina, with millions worldwide engaging in ultramarathons and triathlons in the most exciting and exotic locations. Viewed from an evolutionary point of view, the incredible distances that are covered today only by elite athletes were much more common in ancestral times – just without the energy bars and fanfare.

Central to all this are our legs and our ability to walk upright. Ever since Charles Darwin published *On the Origin of Species* in 1859, researchers have been fascinated by the evolution of man's ability to walk on two legs. Our bipedalism makes us something of a rarity in the animal kingdom, leading anthropologists to question why it is that we favour two legs over four. While there remains debate as to exactly when man made the switch to a hands-free stride, it seems likely that this change happened between four and seven million years ago.

Over time, human anatomy evolved to increase the efficiency of walking upright. This included countless adaptations of our physical body and physiological processes. Many of these changes occurred in the feet, such as reduced stiffness in the midfoot. This seemingly small adaptation encourages us to touch the ground heel-first when walking, which increases our effective leg length and improves walking speed. This 'heel-strike' gait also helps us transition more quickly from walking to running (Webber & Raichlen, 2016).

Taking a single step involves around 400 individual muscles. And while walking requires hardly any active thinking and coordination, the neuronal network, which is responsible for putting one foot in front of the other, is even more impressive. Nevertheless, the omnipresent conveniences of our civilised world, with cars, elevators, and an opportunity to sit down wherever we are, neglect this incredible capability which becomes less of an essential part of our very existence. But this convenience does come at a cost, as we will see.

Walking upright has done more than change the shape and function of our feet, though. Its effects extend to our entire musculoskeletal system, affecting the size, shape, and angle of the pelvis in relation to the spine (Pontzer, 2017). These adaptations have helped create a stable hip joint with a wide range of motion – a structure well-suited to days spent walking in search of food and water (Warrener, 2017), less so than sitting in an office chair for extended hours every day, with the muscles responsible for acting and stabilising the hip joints effectively switched off.

The increase in desk-based jobs over physical labour in the last 150 years or so has given rise to a largely sedentary population across many countries. This change in behaviour has – in the grand scheme of human existence – happened at a much faster pace than would allow for physiological adaptation. The result is an onslaught of conditions that disrupt the natural shape of our musculoskeletal apparatus, leading to millions of debilitating cases of shoulder, neck and back pain, disc herniations, chronic headaches, joint degenerations and more. Virtually all of this suffering is not only unnecessary, but self-inflicted.

The modern world's understanding of a flexible and agile body is today more associated with yoga and lifestyle, than it is to be considered a basic necessity for all. The harsh reality of this fundamental misconception usually only strikes people's own awareness once they find themselves being affected and not able to carry out common tasks efficiently and without external help or pain. In fact, in many parts of the western world, only an artificial construct of caregivers in ambulant and stationary settings enables a growing percentage of our older population to stay alive and engage in everyday life.

The coming chapters shed new light and scientific insight on the most common complications of sitting on the musculoskeletal system and how to avoid them. You might want to take a walk, before reading on.

THE CORE AND THE SPINE – OUR WEAK SPOTS WHEN SITTING

Most of the muscular pain conditions from sitting results from ignorance of our core, which is a normally very well counterbalanced system of muscles, bones and structures that enable the rest of our body to maintain an upright posture when on our feet.

Simply put, after millions of years walking, we now spend most of the day sitting. When we sit – or more often, when we slouch – in a chair with back support, it removes the need for our abdominal muscles to remain active. As these muscles relax, the task of staying upright falls on the spine. The spine and supporting back muscles will do this job for quite a while, and by the time that it begins to cause consistent discomfort, damage has often progressed beyond the point of a cure and long-term pain sets in.

Sitting also changes the angle of the pelvis and hips, which work with the spine to create a strong, stable and upright posture that allows us to manipulate items with our hands, while standing or moving (Labelle et al., 2005; Roussouly & Pinheiro-Franco, 2011).

The spine is normally aligned in an S-like shape. When we begin changing the angle of the pelvis and hips by sitting for extended periods of time, we force the spine out of its usual shape and creating substantial shear forces at critical junctions, most prominent in the area of the cervical spine and lower back. It is by no coincidence that these are the very regions that are most affected by disc herniations and chronic back pain.

HOW TO PROTECT YOUR GLUTES

Among all muscles, the glutes are distinct as we tend to care more about their physical appearance, especially with regard to the perception of our own attractiveness to others and our personal image of ourselves.

Studying the anatomy of the glutes, it becomes immediately clear that these muscle powerhouses were never meant to be squeezed between a chair and the weight of our upper body for hours on end. This starts with the skin. Areas of the body that are genetically designed to be in contact with the ground have a different skin composition. The best example are the soles of our feet, with calluses building up quickly and thick layers of brown fat cells to cushion the repetitive impact from walking. If the gluteal area had been designed to be in constant touch to the ground (or a chair), we would expect to see something comparable – yet nothing could be more different from the delicate skin of our buttocks.

Under the skin of the glutes lies a complicated layer of nerves, blood vessels, muscles, and bones that function in support of holding an upright posture. In actuality, their continuously compressed state does the opposite and comes with its own unique set of issues.

When functioning properly, the glute muscles work with other muscles in the hips to help stabilise the pelvis. When shut off while seated, the body attempts to compensate for the instability through the use of other muscles to keep the pelvis stable. This contributes to lower back and hip pain as the muscles that are in charge to flex the hip joint become tight and constantly pull the lower sections of the spine forward.

After years of abuse from sitting, the glute muscles can be damaged to the point that is referred to 'gluteal amnesia,' casually referred to as the 'dead butt syndrome,' in which those muscles basically forget how to function due to lack of use, resulting in compromised blood flow and nerve damage. Take a moment to wake up your glutes and remind them on a daily basis how much you like and need them!

BACK PAIN – A GLOBAL CRISIS

Back pain seems so universal nowadays, we can almost forget that it is something that affects many of our lives on a daily basis. Spanning all variations and intensities, back pain can range from a mild discomfort to a full immobilising and debilitating state that requires immediate medical care. It is also the leading cause of disability in most countries and across all age groups, with over half a billion people affected worldwide (Hurwitz et al., 2018). Given the ageing population in most countries, and the increase in sedentary behaviour, this trend is likely to only worsen in the years to come.

In the U.S., back pain is the 6th most expensive condition, which accounts for the most lost work days. In 2005, approximately 33 million American adults reportedly suffered from back and neck problems, resulting in absence from the workplace (Chandwani, 2013).

While most cases of back pain resolve within six weeks, up to a quarter of cases lead to chronic conditions that can have a profound effect on one's daily life, and a significant chance of negatively affecting a person's mental and emotional health.

Chronic back pain also has huge economic ramifications, with only half of individuals whose disability persists for over six months returning to work (Anderssen, 1999).

It is hard to put a price tag on this, but a study from the U.S. came up with a scary estimation, which illustrates the socioeconomic catastrophe we find ourselves in today. For a two-year period during 2008-2010, the total national costs related to all causes of chronic back pain amounted to an estimated $187 billion, including both direct medical costs and indirect costs, such as that from lost labour. Per person, this worked out to $37,129 in direct medical costs, including $19,849 for prescription medications (Chandwani, 2013). Outside of the United States, the situation is no less dire, as a study that assessed the direct and indirect costs of low back pain in Australia, Belgium, Japan, Korea, the Netherlands, Sweden and the U.K. between 1997 and 2007 concluded that back pain represents a "substantial burden on society" (Dagenais et al., 2008).

Chronic back pain not only has a major impact on a person's ability to show up for work, it also affects productivity while in the office. In one U.S. study, common pain conditions – which attributed to reduced performance but not workplace absence – resulted in a mean average loss of 5.2 hours of productivity per week (Stewart et al., 2003). When we consider just how many people suffer from chronic back pain, we can only imagine just how many productive hours are lost that go unaccounted for.

Professions that require a large amount of sedentary work time, such as vehicle drivers and office workers, are often at the greatest risk for chronic back injuries. An Israeli study looking at 384 male full-time urban bus drivers found that almost every other driver had experienced lower back pain in the past 12 months (Alperovitch-Najenson et al., 2010). Other studies that looked at over 2,500 office workers, have found that between 33% and 50% of participants had experienced back pain within the last year (Ranasinghe et al., 2011, Celik et al., 2018). These numbers likely don't even sound all that surprising, given what we know from our own experiences in the workplace.

HOW BACK PAIN IS
MAKING US MENTALLY SICK

Chronic back and neck pain also take a significant toll on our mental health and wellbeing, and can lead to 'disuse syndrome.' This term, coined in the 1980s, encapsulates the idea that chronic pain conditions act as a downward spiral, leading to more sedentary behaviour and, as a result, a continual decline in both physical and mental capabilities. The concept of 'use it or lose it' means that chronic back and neck pain can adversely affect a person's social and professional interactions, their sexual health, self-image and self-confidence, recreational activities, parenting or caretaking capacity, and their ability to perform everyday tasks related to personal hygiene, cooking, cleaning and overall quality of life.

These restrictions go on to increase a person's vulnerability to malnutrition and infection. In fact, chronic lower back pain has even been associated with a host of deficits in cognitive function, including impairment of information processing speed and working memory (Schiltenwolf et al., 2017).

With this laundry list of associated ailments, it is no surprise that we also see a high correlation between back pain and depression. A Korean study looking at health records for 7,550 people found that, in general, people with lower back pain were nearly four times more likely to be depressed. Respectively, people with severe depression had an increased risk of lower back pain by nine fold!

This certainly represents something of a chicken-egg scenario. A person who is depressed may have a greater sensitivity to pain and may be less physically active and engaged in other healthy behaviours, while somebody with back pain may also have the same difficulties engaging in regular exercise, particularly if they are suffering from sleep problems and are experiencing social and professional isolation and dissatisfaction, all potentially contributing to depression (Alhowimel et al., 2018). Regardless of whether someone initially suffers from depression or back pain, it can lead to a vicious cycle that can be difficult to get out of.

OPIOIDS: A SHORT-TERM SOLUTION
FOR A LONG-TERM PROBLEM

Patients consulting their physician often favour immediate relief, particularly when they know that physicians have a miraculous tool in their arsenal which promises just that – opioids. As Maslow is famously quoted in the law of the instrument, "If all you have is a hammer, everything looks like a nail." This leads us to today: a quick fix that makes patients happy usually results in them coming back for more, but never actually solves the underlying issue.

The rates of prescription opioids for back pain in the United States has skyrocketed, reaching endemic proportions to the point that it has been called a public health emergency. Compared to most European countries, rates of opioid prescriptions are two to three times higher in the U.S. and Canada (Deyo et al., 2015).

Long-term use of opioids can lead to various side effects. With a vicious cycle of increased drug tolerance, harrowing withdrawals, and greater sensitivity to pain (hyperalgesia), addiction sets in with higher risk of overdose and even death. Other issues related to opioid use include the risk of falls and fractures, as well as depression (Deyo et al., 2015).

Given the risks associated with opioid use, one would assume that there must be significant benefits to prescribing these medications for pain management. However, this is not supported by research, as workers who are prescribed opioids for acute back pain do not return to work more quickly, nor do they have improvements in functional outcomes with opioid use. In fact, there is very little research indicating any real benefit to long-term opioid use in the effective management of back pain (Deyo et al., 2015).

TECHNOLOGICAL EVOLUTION
AND THE HUMAN SPINE

Today we have unprecedented – and seemingly unlimited – access to powerful information and communication technology. This has allowed us a level of engagement and freedom previously unheard of and has brought huge advances for civilisation as a whole. This book will not argue anything against that; if anything, this book only reinforces the fact! The problem is, however, that all this technology may not be entirely in line with the requirements of human anatomy, physiology and ergonomics just yet.

Given this unparalleled influx of personal technology usage, and the fact that the first generation to grow up using smartphones, laptops and tablets is now reaching an age where spinal issues are becoming prevalent, it is not surprising just how much research there is regarding the health impact of our technology habits. Since the year 2000, nearly 3,000 research papers have been published related to health issues specifically as it pertains to smartphone use, for example.

The problem is, when we interact with these devices we are often sitting or stationery and tend to hunch our shoulders and slouch. The greatest side effects are seen, therefore, in the cervical spine, because the acting kinematics are significantly altered once the head is positioned in a forward, bended posture. While a short time in this posture won't hurt by any means, as the saying goes, constant dripping wears the stone. The weight of the head increases the pressure on the cervical spine exponentially when bended forward and it is the accumulating hours we rest in such a position day after day that leads to the recent influx of patients with cervical spine issues and chronic neck pain.

A systematic review published in 2017 looked at results from 15 studies and found that up to 67.8% of people using handheld devices had musculoskeletal complaints, with neck pain being the most common symptom (Xie et al., 2017). Excessive use in young adults points to what we can expect in the years to come, though these rates will likely be even more dramatic in the future. Swedish men 20-24 years old had up to a 200% increase in the likelihood of symptoms in the neck and upper extremities when compared to their older counterparts (Gustafsson et al., 2017).

Postural changes aside, the use of technology affects the body in other ways. For a number of reasons, we tend to hold our breath while texting, which reduces tissue oxygenation and increases muscle tension. Given the overall importance of proper breathing habits for one's health, learning to breathe consistently when using the phone may become something we all just have to learn (Lin et al., 2009). While this false breathing pattern could be relatively easy to correct, the overall compromising effect on sitting and our lungs seems to be a whole different subject, which we must learn to decipher.

Leaving the muscles, bones and joints, in the next chapter we will dive deeper into the human body and uncover how a sedentary lifestyle affects our organs and metabolism on a macroscopic down to a subcellular level.

CHAPTER TWO:
HOW SITTING AFFECTS
THE ORGANS AND METABOLISM

GASPING FOR AIR – YOUR LUNGS IN DISTRESS

Breathing is the essence of life. With every breath, humans inhale around half a litre of air, which mainly fuels the energy production of every single cell. Generally speaking, there are only two main states in which we are reminded just how important breathing is to us.

First, in a very pleasant setting, when deeply breathing in fresh air, for example in an inspiring environment in the middle of nature or while performing yoga or meditation. The immediate and measurable calming effect on the body can have a profound impact and truly demonstrates the power of our lungs and interconnection they have to the rest of our bodies.

Second, in a very unpleasant setting, when we suddenly feel as though we can't breathe as we are used to. This is a state that can quickly turn into a life threatening fight for survival and cause uncomfortable arousal.

There is a state in between these two extremes – one which we don't tend to notice because we have gotten so used to it. This is the effect that sitting has on our lungs. While not killing us right away, the long-term effects on our health are outright scary.

It's not uncommon for the average office worker to spend several hours a day in a position in which he or she slumps over a desk with hunched shoulders and a rounded spine. For many, this is a daily norm. While we have become perfectly used to this, and might even appreciate the apparent comfort that comes from this low effort posture, for the lungs it is a highly unnatural state that results in a substantial reduction in oxygen volume.

To understand the whole picture of compression caused by poor posture, it is essential to understand how our lungs work. The lungs are basically just a tissue in which the exchange of air is taking place. Lungs don't have the function to contract or expand by themselves, they just follow the movements of the muscles that surround them. First and foremost, the lungs inflate due to the compression of the underlying diaphragm muscles, which separate the lungs from the lower part of our upper body that contains our stomach and intestines. Breathing primarily happens by moving this layer of muscles down, with the lungs passively following. Only after this first motion do our lungs expand with our rib cage and we inhale fresh air. This second mechanism typically requires intentional action; for example, when engaging in physical exercise we require a greater oxygen intake. In the described typical sedentary posture, the abdominal compartment below the diaphragm is compressed between the upper body and the flexed hip. In this state, our primary breathing mechanism becomes chronically impaired, with the involved muscles losing strength over time. This can lead to something we will get to know shortly as superficial breathing (Landers et al., 2003; Crosbie & Myles, 1985).

While most of us have become used to the diminished lung capacity fostered by poor posture and hardly notice any real difference in our breathing while sitting, some individuals are acutely aware of how posture affects their breath. In a study that looked at the effects of different postures on breathing in brass instrument players, simply sitting down reduced activity in the muscles of the abdominal wall by 32-44% compared to standing. Even sitting on a downward sloping seat led to an 11% reduction in the maximum duration of a note played on a trumpet (Price et al., 2014).

While most of us do not need to worry about holding a note while playing a wind instrument, that does not make us immune to the negative effects of sitting when it comes to our respiratory function. In a study involving 70 able-bodied volunteers, researchers looked at how four different seating positions influenced breathing and lumbar lordosis (the inward curvature of our lower spinal cord). Compared to standing, seated positions were overall worse for lung capacity and expiratory flow, as well as lumbar lordosis. The worst position, associated with significant decreases across all measures, was a slumped posture where the pelvis was positioned in the middle of the seat as the volunteer leaned against a back-rest (Lin et al., 2006). This is exactly the position associated with the typical desk setting.

So why is all this a problem for us? As reduced respiratory function further compromises muscle activity, and as impaired muscle function negatively impacts breathing, this creates something of a vicious circle leading to shallow breathing patterns becoming the norm (Wirth et al., 2014). Taking shallower breaths means less oxygen is delivered to the body's tissue, which compromises cellular metabolism and muscle function, and can lead to decreased stamina and energy.

A lack of oxygen also affects brain activity, and can lead to poor concentration, impaired focus and reduced memory. A reduction in expiratory flow also means that the body is less able to dispel waste gases, including carbon dioxide.

Poorer respiratory function has also been associated with increased levels of stress hormones, whereas deeper, fuller breaths appear to have a calming effect on both the mind and the body. In one study, healthy volunteers who received training in diaphragmatic breathing showed improvements in sustained attention, as well as lower levels of cortisol (the stress hormone) after 20 sessions over eight weeks (Ma et al., 2017).

In recent years, medical research has revealed even more profound impacts on long-term health, specifically the increased risk for cardiovascular disease and stroke (Hancox et al., 2007). This is likely caused by a dysfunction in the smaller blood vessels of the brain when lung capacity is compromised, resulting in a permanently low level inflammatory state. Evidence for this link has been seen in a longitudinal study that assessed respiratory function and cerebral small-vessel disease in women over a period of 26 years. The researchers found that lower scores on two measures of lung function spanning a time frame of 20 years were associated with a higher prevalence and severity of brain lesions and the most common type of stroke (Guo et al., 2006). Other studies looking at respiratory function and cerebrovascular disease have found similar associations, which suggests that improving lung capacity may have a protective effect against stroke in later life (Liao et al., 1999).

Today we are learning that, in addition to being a symptom of cardiovascular disease itself, a chronic shallow breathing pattern may be an independent risk factor for poor cardiovascular health. This association was first noted in the Framingham study, which followed 5,200 individuals over three decades (Sorlie et al., 1989; Ashley et al., 1975) and has been recently followed up in research from Korea, corroborating the idea that improved respiratory function may help decrease a person's risk of cardiovascular disease down the line (Kang et al., 2015).

DIABETES – THE SILENT PANDEMIC

An estimated 422 million people worldwide are affected by diabetes, with the global prevalence of the disease growing exponentially between 1980 and 2014 (from 4.7% to 8.5% of the global population). In 2015 alone, an estimated 1.6 million deaths were directly caused by diabetes. That's equivalent to the entire country of Bahrain succumbing to the complications of the disease in a single year.

America is particularly hard hit by this disease. According to the American

Diabetes Association (ADA) there are over 30 million children and adults living with diabetes in the United States (around 9.4% of the population), with 1.5 million new cases diagnosed each year. While this means that many are likely unaware of their condition, it also serves to normalise the disease, which may result in lowered action or accountability.

Countless individuals are living with undiagnosed diabetes or prediabetes which, if left untreated, will in most cases have serious health effects as the disease progresses. Indeed, diabetes is a leading cause of death and disability, and is listed as the underlying cause or contributing factor in over 250,000 deaths each year in America alone. However, the actual toll of diabetes is likely to be much higher, with recent research showing that, in up to 60% of cases, the death certificates for those with diabetes do not even mention the disease (source ADA).

AN ECONOMIC TSUNAMI

The economic cost of diabetes is staggering. So much so, that the Canadian Diabetes Association (CDA) published a report in 2009 calling diabetes an 'Economic Tsunami.' The CDA predicts that by 2020 a new person will be diagnosed with diabetes every hour of every day.

The economic cost associated with diabetes in the U.S. provides a forecast of what lies ahead for many economies in the decades to come. In the U.S., direct medical costs of treatment for diabetes amounted to $176 billion in 2010, with losses in productivity reaching another $69 billion. Worldwide, estimates from a recent systematic review put the direct annual cost of diabetes at around $827 billion (Seuring et al., 2015). The International

Diabetes Federation (IDF) estimates that total global healthcare spending on diabetes has more than tripled between 2003 and 2013 (IDF, 2013).

In recent years, the prevalence of diabetes has been rising more rapidly in middle- and low-income countries, meaning that some of the poorest communities will be forced to address an unprecedented economic and societal burden. One study estimated that from 2011-2030, losses in gross domestic product (GDP) will total $1.7 trillion worldwide, with $800 billion of that shouldered by those in low- and middle-income brackets (Bloom et al., 2011). And all this for a disease that is largely preventable.

WHAT IS DIABETES AND HOW DOES IT DEVELOP?

Despite being a very common disease, there is still widespread confusion around what diabetes actually is, and perhaps even more confusion around the different types. Simply speaking, diabetes is a chronic condition resulting from the body's inability to sufficiently produce or properly use insulin, the hormone that enables sugar to be transported into cells to produce energy.

There are two types of diabetes, as well as prediabetes, a condition where blood sugar is higher than normal but not yet high enough for a diagnosis. Having prediabetes increases the risk of developing diabetes itself, as well as the risk of cardiovascular disease and neuropathy.

Type 1 diabetes is an autoimmune disease that often arises in childhood.

Type 2 diabetes, the most common form, can occur in children and adults and is typically related to lifestyle and diet.

Type 2 diabetes was previously referred to as 'adult-onset diabetes' (or non-insulin dependent diabetes, NIDDM), but poor diet and increasingly sedentary behaviour early in life means that millions of children will develop this 'adult' disease, and with it some serious health consequences.

In addition to sitting for hours each day at school, children are more likely than ever before to eschew outdoor play and physical activity. Instead, most children now spend their free time watching television, playing video games, and using computers or smartphones while sitting. In North America, children and teenagers spend 40-60% of their waking hours engaged in some form of screen-time pursuits (Saunders et al., 2014). And they are becoming used to and dependant on these devices at ever earlier ages; today, it is all too common to see toddlers confidently maneuvering their parents' smartphones.

All this sedentary behaviour, combined with poor diet and an increased risk of having had a mother with diabetes, dramatically increases a child's risk of developing type 2 diabetes later in life, if not in childhood itself (WHO, 2016). Type 2 diabetes, the 'adult' disease of modern civilisation, is now seen in children as young as six years old (Diabetes UK, 2010).

The prevalence of type 2 diabetes is increasing around the world in children of all ethnicities. While it is strongly associated with obesity, this disease can also manifest in children who are of a normal weight and may be asymptomatic or only display mild symptoms, which can delay diagnosis and treatment thereby increasing the risk of serious health effects.

In type 2 diabetes, the pancreas may produce too little insulin, and the liver might overproduce glucose, resulting in elevated blood sugar. The main problem, though, is peripheral insulin resistance, particularly in muscle cells.

Our bodies need insulin to effectively use sugar as an energy source. When we do not have enough insulin, or when our cells become insulin-resistant, the sugar in our blood is unable to enter cells. This means that our blood sugar levels rise, and our cells are deprived of the fuel they need to function correctly. As a result, symptoms of diabetes can include unwanted weight loss, fatigue, slow and impaired healing and immune function, cognitive deficits, and a whole host of other issues resulting from a general diminishing of normal and healthy physiological processes.

THE COMPLICATIONS FROM DIABETES

When blood glucose levels remain elevated, the same glucose that fuels our cells and maintains energy production begins to act as toxin on the vessels, resulting in pathological changes in organs including the eyes, nerves, kidneys, brain and blood vessels, respectively. Poorly managed or untreated diabetes can consequently lead to cardiovascular disease, stroke, kidney failure, neuropathy, retinopathy, blindness and lower limb amputations.

The risk associated with diabetes for cardiovascular disease is profound. An individual with diabetes is at the same risk of cardiovascular disease as someone (without diabetes) who has previously suffered a heart attack. Diabetes also doubles the risk of stroke in the first five years following diagnosis, compared to the general population (Diabetes UK, 2010).

In the U.S., almost 40% of adults with diabetes will develop chronic kidney disease, and in 2014 over 50,000 people required dialysis after being diagnosed with end-stage kidney disease (WHO, 2016). Diabetes is the single most common cause of kidney failure, or end-stage renal disease, worldwide. Kidney disease accounts for 21% of deaths in type 1 diabetes and 11% of deaths in type 2 diabetes (Department of Health, 2007; Morrish et al., 2001).

It goes without saying that kidney disease can dramatically affect the quality of one's life, necessitating the use of medications and regular dialysis. What's more, having diabetes often means that the affected patient may be a poor candidate for a kidney transplant, due to an increased risk of infection and other complications.

Another real threat is the risk of losing one's eyesight, as diabetes is a leading cause of blindness (Diabetes UK, 2010; CDA, 2009). Persistently elevated blood sugar levels leads to damage in the retina, optic nerve and blood vessels. Within 20 years of being diagnosed, 60% of people with type 2 diabetes will have some degree of retinopathy (Scanlon, 2008). Diabetes also doubles the risk of other debilitating eye diseases, such as cataracts and glaucoma (Petit & Adamec, 2002).

Given the host of associated ailments noted above, it's not surprising that many diabetes patients also suffer from depression (CDA, 2009). This is likely due to a combination of the symptoms of the disease itself, difficulties posed by managing it (such as financial and familial burden) and biochemical factors (Kiecolt-Glaser, 2015).

Taken together, the average diabetes patient can expect to lose 10-20 years of their life expectancy. This fact alone shows just how important it is to take preventative steps to curb the risk for diabetes, which can be achieved with some simple lifestyle changes including diet and exercise.

HOW SITTING INCREASES
YOUR RISK OF DIABETES

Inactivity and sedentariness are the greatest risk factors for developing diabetes. Even somebody with an unfavourable dietary pattern might be able to get away with it, but it doesn't work the other way around. In most cases, the combination of a poor diet with a job that includes long hours seated create the perfect metabolic storm.

Data from a large Brazilian study supports this idea. Researchers looked at over 60,000 men and women and found that watching television for more than four hours a day was associated with a 64% higher incidence of type 2 diabetes in men and a whopping 96% higher incidence of heart disease, with only slightly less dramatic numbers for women (Werneck et al., 2018).

Why is being sedentary such a big deal for diabetes? Physical activity improves how our cells respond to insulin which, in turn, improves our body's ability to regulate blood glucose. Physical activity also supports better blood lipids, blood pressure and activity of the fat-burning enzyme lipoprotein lipase, which is key to understanding the implications of sitting and the rise of diabetes (more on that shortly). Finally, physical activity also helps with stress management and weight management, which is important because these are two known risk factors for diabetes in their own right.

Experimental studies have shown that prolonged sitting, with a respective reduction in the contraction of the large leg muscles, suppresses insulin activity and the activity of muscle lipoprotein lipase (LPL). LPL is an enzyme found primarily on the surface of cells that line tiny blood vessels in muscles and fatty tissue, and is essential for the breakdown of triglycerides (a form of fat) for use as energy. This is why muscle LPL levels are typically higher in athletes, as they need the LPL to replenish the muscle energy stores after exercise (Seip et al., 1998).

When muscle LPL activity is low, triglycerides are either stored in fat cells or remain in the blood, as opposed to being used for energy. Higher circulating levels of triglycerides increase the risk of cardiovascular disease, while a higher percentage of body fat increases insulin resistance. People with lower muscle LPL activity and higher LPL activity in fatty tissue are more likely to gain weight, particularly unhealthy body fat, compared to people with greater LPL activity in muscles (Ferland et al., 2012). Even people who have low muscle LPL activity and high LPL activity in fatty tissue, but are not obese or even overweight, are at a higher risk of diabetes, cardiovascular disease and metabolic syndrome. This is because so-called 'thin-outside-fat-inside' people carry a higher amount of visceral fat around their organs in the abdomen, which increases insulin resistance as well as the production of inflammatory cytokines (Thomas et al., 2012).

Regular long lasting activities, such as walking or biking, are particularly effective in maintaining a high level of LPL activity in slow-twitch postural skeletal muscles, whereas higher intensity exercise, such as running or tennis, is important for LPL activity in fast-twitch glycolytic muscles. As we age, we typically see a reduction in LPL activity in skeletal muscle fibres. A comparable pattern of reduced LPL activity is also seen in sedentary people. Interestingly, even older adults who engage in endurance training have been found to have a better blood lipid profile than younger sedentary adults (Hamilton et al., 2001). This just goes to show that, regardless of your age, it's not too late to start incorporating new habits that can dramatically change your health and wellbeing.

Studies show that muscle LPL activity increases with even light exercise, compared to when sitting (Hamilton et al., 2007), but will not persist after the activity ends. This underscores the notion that a human truly needs to be engaged in low intensity movement regularly throughout the day in order to maintain a healthy metabolism (Bey et al., 2003).

PREVENTING AND REVERSING DIABETES

For people at risk, physical activity and modest weight loss have been shown to lower the risk of type 2 diabetes by up to 58%. The difficulty is, when your cells aren't getting enough fuel it can feel like an impossible battle to go for even a quick run around the block.

Instead of focusing on the occasional bouts of intense exercise, the best way to prevent, delay or manage diabetes is simply to stop sitting and start walking. Taking a stroll after breakfast, lunch and dinner has been shown to prevent the postprandial (post-meal) spike in blood glucose, as well as lower blood pressure. Those after-meal blood sugar spikes pose a significant risk for cardiometabolic disease but can be greatly reduced by cutting back on sitting time. A walk immediately following a meal has been proven to contribute to a significant reduction in blood glucose. One study showed that blood glucose was decreased by nearly 50% when meals were followed by walking, both in healthy individuals as well as those with type 1 diabetes (Manohar et al., 2012). While true for everybody, people with diabetes or those who are at risk should carefully avoid prolonged sitting times and search for ways to incorporate more movement during the day. It could make all the difference in the world (Dempsey et al., 2018).

In an evolutionary context, the release of blood glucose as a response to a stressful stimuli makes complete sense, as this boost of fast available energy was often essential for survival. In today's world, however, many of us have no physical release for stress in the workplace, meaning that stress caused by workload and looming deadlines is most likely dealt with while remaining seated. So, while the way we spend our days has changed dramatically over the past few thousand years, our bodies' response to stress has not and release of the stress hormone cortisone still triggers the same elevation in blood glucose as it did in our prehistoric ancestors. Upon identifying a stressor, our bodies immediately flood with adrenaline and norepinephrine, which increases our heart rate and respiration, causes sweating, and gives us a surge of energy that allows us to focus our attention and flee from danger. Cortisol takes a little bit longer to kick in (minutes versus seconds) because it requires a rather lengthy chain of actors in the brain and the kidneys to be activated before cortisol is released. Since the body is in rescue mode at this time, it will also temporarily silence all non-emergency systems, such as the reproductive system, digestive system, growth and immune functions. Most importantly, in the context of diabetes, storage of blood glucose in cells is not desirable in an emergency setting, which makes cortisol a very potent antagonist of insulin. While measures to counterbalance stress span a wide range of possibilities and are beyond the scope of this book, a simple reduction in sitting time will ensure that the available energy has a place to be used when it comes into play.

Perhaps the linchpin of reducing the risk of diabetes is weight management. The problem with being overweight is that it decreases insulin sensitivity itself, creating another vicious cycle with huge implications for health, as we will see in more detail further on.

WHAT SITTING MEANS FOR THE HEART

A heart attack is the ultimate complication of a disease, which may often remain silent for years before revealing itself in a single, and sometimes deadly event. Heart disease remains the number one cause of deaths worldwide, accounting for more than 15 million deaths in 2015 alone. In comparison, road injuries killed 1.3 million people in the same year (WHO, 2017). According to the American Heart Association, up to 80% of heart disease and strokes are preventable. So, what exactly happens to the heart during an attack?

With every beat, the heart sends a portion of blood through a range of blood vessels in order to nurture and fuel itself. As a powerful muscle in constant action, the heart has a steady demand for oxygen and nutrients.

These rather tiny blood vessels of the heart are called the coronary arteries. With diameters in the millimetre range, the coronary arteries are at a much higher risk of becoming clotted. These clots arise through gradual build-up on the vessel walls until they eventually rupture and a blood clot forms on its surface. As the clot grows, it can become large enough that it blocks circulation to parts of the heart, leading to a heart attack. Comparable blood clots can also form in other damaged blood vessels throughout the body, and if these dislodge and travel to smaller blood vessels, such as in the brain or lungs, it can result in stroke or pulmonary embolism. The underlying process is often the same.

How does a sedentary lifestyle contribute to this pathology? Why is sitting too much becoming even more dangerous to our cardiac health than smoking, as is often cited in current headlines?

In its essence, heart disease can be understood as a metabolic disease, where an unfavourable mixture of biochemicals plaque the blood vessels over an extended period of time. The lack of movement that comes along with being sedentary promotes this unfavourable mix in the blood and body. It can also increase the risk of heart attack or stroke by reducing healthy blood flow, weakening the heart muscle, which in turn raises blood pressure and creates a permanent low-level inflammatory state.

Sedentary behaviour also makes it more likely that a person will gain unhealthy body fat and lose lean muscle mass. As discussed in the last chapter, weight gain can lead to insulin resistance and impair blood glucose regulation, while increasing levels of circulating triglycerides and low-density lipoprotein (LDL) cholesterol. High blood pressure also puts extra strain on the blood vessels and heart, all leading to damage and possible consequent plaque formation. Being physically active helps keep the blood glucose in check and is one of the best things one can do to raise levels of beneficial high-density lipoprotein (HDL) cholesterol, which helps to clear LDL cholesterol from your arteries.

The scientific data from the last ten years or so can easily be distilled to a single message: the more hours somebody spends sitting each day, the higher his or her likelihood for getting diagnosed with some form of heart disease later on in life, regardless of whether the person is otherwise active in his or her leisure time. Here are some of the most impressive data.

In one study looking at almost a quarter of a million adults aged 50-71, those who spent seven or more hours a day sitting, compared to those who sat for less than one hour a day, had an 85% increased risk of death from cardiovascular disease (Matthews et al., 2012). Other studies have shown that people who sit a lot have a much higher risk of high blood pressure (a 71% increase in one study), as well as being 42% more likely to have lower levels of beneficial high-density lipoprotein (HDL) cholesterol (Park et al., 2018). Interestingly, this study also found that no amount of intense exercise was able to make up for all that sitting: people who spent seven or more hours a day sitting also had twice the risk of death from cardiovascular disease, even if they also spent one or more hours a day exercising (Matthews et al., 2012). Statistically, for every two hours a person spent sitting each day, the risk for cardiovascular disease increases by an additional 5% (Ford & Casperson, 2012).

Once affected by a heart attack or another cardiac disease, patients often have a significantly reduced quality of life, experiencing associated symptoms such as shortness of breath, fatigue and reduced physical capacity, making exercise increasingly difficult and resulting in more hours spent sedentary.

On the other hand, for a long time cardiologists have proclaimed that long-term low to moderate physical activity (such as walking) appears to have an overall favourable effect on one's cardiovascular health.

One of the largest studies looked at more than a million people and compared their walking behaviour with their risk of being diagnosed with heart disease. It seems as though walking can have miraculous effects on the heart. People who walked around an hour each day or around 20km per week could lower their heart risk by almost a third (Hamer & Chida, 2014). That is better than what so many medications on the market could ever hope to provide, and instead of side effects, walking comes with side benefits! Other studies have pointed to similarly promising findings. Simply incorporating daily walking time led to a 29% lowered risk of hypertension in over 6,000 Japanese men (Hayashi et al., 1999), and a 27% lowered mortality rate in 2,000 Americans with just four hours of walking per week (LaCroix et al., 1996).

IS SITTING PREVENTING
YOU FROM LOSING WEIGHT?

More people are overweight or obese than ever before, prompting the World Health Organization to acknowledge this as a 'Globesity' epidemic. The number of people worldwide who are overweight (BMI higher than 25) or obese (BMI higher than 30) has skyrocketed in recent years, from an estimated 200 million adults in 1995 to over 300 million as of 2000 (WHO press release, 2003). Data from a recent analysis of 188 countries suggests that the number has risen even further in the last decade, with more than a third of adults qualifying as overweight (Ng et al., 2014). In some countries more than half of all men and women are obese. As adults over the age of

15 account for around 75% of the world's population, this suggests that there are now an astonishing 2.12 billion adults worldwide who are overweight.

Even more worrying is the fact that the prevalence of overweight and obesity increased by nearly 50% in children and adolescents between 1980 and 2013. As of 2013, more than one in five girls and nearly one in four boys living in developed countries were overweight, as were more than one in eight children in developing countries (Ng et al., 2014). Children who are overweight have reduced lifespan, and are at a high risk of spending their lives living with disability.

In 2010, an estimated three to four million deaths were attributed to being overweight or obese, with people losing 3-9% of their projected lifespan to these conditions (Ng et al., 2014). Being overweight significantly increases a person's risk of cardiovascular disease, diabetes, joint issues, back pain, cancer, hypertension and premature death. Beyond the physical implications, weight can also have a major effect on a person's sense of wellbeing and happiness, with several studies showing higher levels of depression in those who are obese, including one recent analysis of data from over 9,000 adults in the U.S. (Simon et al., 2006).

THE ECONOMIC AND SOCIETAL COSTS OF OBESITY

Obesity is a complex condition with serious consequences for society and the individual. It affects people regardless of age, race, gender, or socioeconomic group, and costs a staggering amount of money in healthcare and lost productivity. In 2014, the worldwide economic impact of obesity was estimated to be USD $2.0 trillion, or 2.8% of the global gross domestic product (GDP) (Dobbs et al., 2014). In the U.S. alone, the annual healthcare costs associated with obesity amount to an estimated $147-210 billion each year, with additional costs of around $4.3 billion from absenteeism (Cawley & Meyerhoefer, 2012; Cawley et al., 2007).

Because obesity itself is not a disease, it is difficult to accurately discern the associated costs. However, it is abundantly clear that increasing BMI is associated with rising healthcare costs to the individual, employers, governments, and societies at large.

Obesity describes the accumulation of fat to a point where it becomes a risk factor for chronic diseases. A person who is overweight has an increased risk of:

- Type 2 diabetes
- Hypertension (high blood pressure)
- Heart disease and heart attack
- Stroke
- Several types of cancer
- Kidney disease
- Non-alcoholic fatty liver disease (NAFLD)
- Sleep apnea
- Osteoarthritis
- Complications in pregnancy, including hypertension, gestational diabetes, and increased risk for cesarean delivery (C-section)

In one study that looked at diseases in adults in South Africa, 68% of hypertensive disease, 45% of ischemic stroke, 38% of ischemic heart disease, and 87% of type 2 diabetes could be attributed to being overweight or obese (Joubert et al., 2007).

Being overweight also raises an individual's risk of at least thirteen types of cancer, which we'll look at more closely towards the end of this chapter.

Non-alcoholic fatty liver disease (NAFLD), liver fibrosis and cirrhosis of the liver, are all associated with obesity. Typically, liver disease, which includes fat accumulation in the liver, is the result of alcohol misuse, but NAFLD has become increasingly common as obesity rates continue to climb. Indeed, NAFLD is now the second most common reason for liver transplants and is the underlying cause of a significant number of liver cancers (Fabbrini et al., 2010; Marchesini et al., 2008; Younossi & Henry, 2015).

Carrying excess body weight also increases pressure on the joints and the spine, leading to degeneration of connective tissue, spinal discs, and bones. Accordingly, being overweight or obese increases the risk of joint pain, back pain, and sciatica (pain that radiates from the sciatic nerve, running from the lower spine down to the foot). This is not surprising, given that degeneration in the intervertebral discs and joints of the spine can lead to spinal stenosis (narrowing of the spaces in the spine) and compression of the sciatic nerve.

Individuals who are overweight can start to see significant positive changes in their body composition, insulin sensitivity, inflammation levels, and a variety of other health risk factors by simply sitting less and walking more. Before we look at how walking can support healthy weight management, let's quickly examine another, lesser known barrier to weight loss: the reduced action of leptin and insulin and their effects on the neurotransmitter dopamine.

HOW SITTING MANIPULATES HORMONES AND AFFECTS APPETITE

Metabolic hormones, such as leptin and insulin play a key role in regulating energy metabolism, in part by acting on the central nervous system, specifically the hypothalamus in the brain. The hypothalamus controls a significant portion of the body's hormonal (endocrine) system through the pituitary gland. In addition to helping regulate energy expenditure and storage, the hypothalamus also plays a role in controlling body temperature, appetite and digestion, and even our circadian rhythms.

The hypothalamus gathers information about short-term energy supply, satiety, and hunger via the vagus nerve that connects the brain to the gut. It also gathers information about long-term energy storage and helps us to recognise when we need to consume more calories for future exertion and longer term survival. Incredibly, just two hormones, leptin and insulin, provide this key information to the hypothalamus to help maintain energy homeostasis. We've already mentioned insulin and its effects on metabolism, so let's turn our attention to the second hormone, leptin.

Leptin (from the Greek, leptos, meaning thin) was first discovered in 1994 in obese mice. It is a small protein that is created in fat cells (adipocytes); the more body fat a person has, the higher their blood leptin levels. If ghrelin is the 'hunger hormone,' leptin is the opposite, telling the brain – specifically the hypothalamus – when we have stored enough energy and no longer need to consume calories. In a healthy system, gastric distension (stretching of the stomach) after a meal results in a signal being sent via the vagus nerve (the gut-brain axis) prompting the release of leptin from fat stores. When leptin crosses the blood-brain barrier and reaches the hypothalamus, it triggers the brain to suppress appetite and increase physical activity.

After it was discovered, leptin attracted the attention of many pharmaceutical companies who considered it the holy grail for weight management. These companies poured huge amounts of money into research and manufacturing leptin-based supplements, but the hormone would never achieve the anticipated success, leaving researchers scratching their heads. What went wrong? Why didn't leptin live up to its early promise as a weight management tool?

The short answer is that the problem isn't leptin deficiency, but rather leptin resistance, i.e. it's not the amount of leptin in the blood that matters, but how well the brain responds to it.

Leptin deficiency is actually very rare and results from either a genetic mutation, brain trauma, or brain surgery. Without proper treatment, people with leptin deficiencies typically become obese and experience other significant and related health issues. The administration of leptin in leptin deficient people serves to normalise their appetite and energy homeostasis, helping them achieve healthier body weights. Leptin resistant individuals, however, do not respond to the administration of supplemental leptin, hence the frustration of those pharmaceutical giants.

EXPERIENCING FALSE HUNGER

There's been plenty of discussion surrounding insulin resistance in recent years, but very little when it comes to leptin resistance. This phenomenon is becoming increasingly common and is most often seen in people who are obese and/or sedentary. In a state of leptin resistance, an individual has high blood levels of leptin (corresponding to a high degree of body fat), but the brain fails to respond to the hormone. This prompts the brain to send out alarm signals telling the body that it is starving and that the person should eat as many calories as possible in order to survive. At the same time, the brain is also telling the body to conserve as much energy as possible, in part by – you guessed it! – being more sedentary. The hypothalamus responds via the vagus nerve to prompt the release of more insulin from the pancreas, further compounding the issue by increasing the risk of insulin resistance.

In a healthy system, insulin production increases after a meal so that the body can transport glucose from the blood into cells for use as energy. When a person is resistant to leptin, this leads to chronic increases in insulin as part of the body's attempt to store more and more energy (Kolaczynski et al., 1996). Insulin also appears to block leptin receptors in the brain, creating a cyclical problem (Imbeault et al., 2001).

By default, the body's system is set to store and conserve energy, a process which served us well in the past. From an evolutionary point of view, storing energy in fat cells was crucial for survival as it helped our ancestors maintain their strength and survive for longer when food was scarce and calorie intake irregular.

However, given that most of us have almost constant access to high calorie food, a system that is set to store fat and encourage us to keep eating can rapidly lead to dramatic weight gain.

In people with leptin resistance, not only is the body sending out panic signals telling them to keep eating, it also acts via the sympathetic nervous system to tip the body into conservation mode, promoting lower energy expenditure and physical activity. And the comfort of the office chair provides just that. This is one of the reasons why people with diabetes, as well as those who are inactive and/or overweight, are more likely to experience depression and greater effects from stress and lethargy.

Leptin also follows a circadian rhythm that is in direct opposition to the daily peaks and troughs of cortisol, the 'stress hormone' (Froy, 2010). Levels of leptin drop in the morning (prompting us to eat), reach their lowest point around noon, and then rise in the evening to reach their highest after midnight. In contrast, cortisol levels are typically highest in the morning and drop in the evening, helping us feel active during the day and relax at night. Poor stress management and a disturbed circadian rhythm can wreak havoc on our natural leptin cycle. This explains why it can be harder to manage appetite if we experience sleep deprivation, work night shifts, have jet lag, or are exposed to blue light from screens and interior lighting after the sun has set. For many, this will sound all too familiar. Furthermore, this disruption explains why appetite and motivation can suffer when we experience a high level of daily stress with no opportunity for an adequate physical response, i.e. no chance for fight or flight. And the situation only becomes more dire as, the next day, the cycle continues.

In recent years, researchers have discovered that leptin doesn't solely engage the hypothalamus for energy homeostasis. The hormone also interacts with the dopaminergic system in the brain. Dopamine has many functions and is our main 'reward' neurotransmitter, driving motivation and willpower. Dopamine also plays an important role in memory, focus and mood. Dysfunction in the dopaminergic system can lead to neurodegeneration, mood disorders, and is associated with psychiatric conditions such as schizophrenia. The dopamine pathway is also the main target in drug addiction.

Leptin also has a role to play in the dopaminergic system, by promoting balance. When it is functioning correctly, leptin signals to the brain that we have enough energy, from either food intake or fat reserves. It does this by extinguishing the dopaminergic reward pathway. However, this mechanism does not work properly in a person with leptin resistance, which means that they are driven to continually seek more rewards by consuming; for many this means more sugary or fatty foods. This same mechanism is at work in drug addiction, where brain dopamine receptors become desensitised over time, prompting the individual to seek increasingly intense stimuli to achieve the same level of reward response.

YOUR BRAIN ON DOPAMINE – WHO'S IN CHARGE?

Beyond maintaining a healthy level of food intake, dopamine is also key to regulating physical activity. Damage and dysfunction in the dopamine system have been linked to movement disorders such as Parkinson's disease, as well as to addictive behaviour, depression, and sedentary behaviour. Dysfunctional dopamine receptors lead to anergia, i.e. a shift to low effort options for reward. This has been demonstrated in animals, with studies showing that mice with depleted dopamine levels spend less time engaged in high-effort exercise activities (like running in a wheel) and are instead more likely to choose low-effort rewards such as sucrose treats (López-Cruz et al., 2018). Post-mortem studies of brains of individuals who were overweight have also revealed significant dysfunction in the dopaminergic system, leading researchers to suggest that a dopamine reward deficiency syndrome may underlie abnormal eating and exercise behaviour that can lead to obesity (Wu et al., 2017).

In recent years, researchers have found that a certain kind of dopamine receptor (D2) in the basal ganglia area of the brain is less active in those who are overweight (Ruegsegger & Booth, 2017) and continued weight gain seems to progressively dull D2 dopamine receptor activity (Kravitz et al., 2016). In practice, this means that an overweight person is less likely to experience 'runner's high' – the pleasurable reward response many people feel during and following exercise – which means they may feel less inclined to begin exercise in the first place.

It is important to distinguish that reduced sensitivity to dopamine does not cause a person to gain weight. Rather, the state of being overweight may make people feel less motivation to exercise, leading to a further sedentary lifestyle and increased weight gain. Another vicious cycle. Less exercise leads to more weight gain, more leptin resistance, and more dopamine receptor dysfunction, all which further decreases our motivation to stop sitting and start moving. Once you understand the underlying mechanisms at play, it's not hard to see how a person who is mostly sedentary can enter into a downward spiral resulting in obesity and a host of associated issues.

There is also evidence that exercise-induced increases in dopamine signalling can lead to increases in brain-derived neurotrophic factor (BDNF), which we will discuss at length in the next chapter. This protein supports healthy neuron growth in the brain, maintaining what is called neuroplasticity. Basically, BDNF helps the brain rewire itself, so we can continue to learn new things and stay flexible in our thinking. Part of this includes helping us better regulate our appetites and adopt healthier dietary and lifestyle habits for successful weight management (Ferris et al., 2007; Pelleymounter at al., 1995).

These recent insights into the dopaminergic system strongly suggest that it's unfair to assume that overweight individuals all just lack the willpower and motivation to exercise more and eat less. Instead, it appears increasingly likely that the brain itself can scupper our best intentions by making exercise seem like far too much effort for far too little reward. These same changes in the brain may make it more likely for us to derive greater pleasure from things that require little effort, such as eating foods high in sugar and fat and seeking comfort by spending the day off our feet (Ruegsegger & Booth, 2017).

The good news is that exercise not only helps enhance insulin sensitivity for improved energy metabolism, it can also make the brain better respond to dopamine. Switching sedentary behaviour for physical activity helps to increase dopamine receptor availability in people with D2 receptor dysfunction, actually making them more likely to want to keep exercising (Robertson et al., 2016). Regular exercise, a healthy diet, and moderate weight loss can help 'reboot' dopamine receptors. This leads to improvements in dopamine levels and dopamine response, helping people who are overweight actually enjoy exercise, while simultaneously supporting improved appetite regulation. Now this is a good cycle to fall into!

SHOULD WE JUST WALK MORE?

Based on a number of studies, the short answer is a resounding yes. First off, walking creates a great opportunity for breaking out of this de-motivation trap. One study found that people with early stages of Parkinson's disease (a condition characterised by decreased dopamine) who walked on a treadmill three times a week for eight weeks had improvements in dopamine receptor response compared to patients who didn't use the treadmills (Fisher et al., 2013).

Not only is low-intensity exercise, such as walking, effective for supporting insulin sensitivity and overall energy metabolism, it also appears to enhance our ability to feel good about making healthier lifestyle choices. Good decisions yield good decisions. Walking is also a good choice for many because it puts less strain on the joints than other more intense forms of exercise. This means that people are less likely to experience walking-related injuries that hinder their attempts to lose weight through exercise.

Studies show that most of us gain around one kg (2.2 lbs) a year in middle-age. While this may not initially seem like a huge difference, it quickly adds up over time! Luckily, we are able to avoid most of this weight gain by walking more. The protective effect of walking has even been seen in people who don't perform other types of exercise, i.e. people who just walk are more likely to avoid weight gain in middle age compared to those who hit the gym a few times a week but are otherwise sedentary. (Gordon-Larsen et al., 2009).

Today, it is abundantly clear that walking can be a great way to break free from the vicious cycle outlined above and instead create a positive feedback loop that supports healthy weight management, better cardiovascular and cognitive health, and a generally happier outlook on life.

WALKING THE WEIGHT AWAY

For anyone struggling to lose excess body weight and get into a positive exercise routine, it helps to start out small and gradually integrate more movement into daily life. This might mean going for a short (15 minute) brisk walk after meals.

The aim should be to increase walking time by 1,000-1,500 steps a day (something most people can achieve in around 15 minutes), and build up to 15,000 steps daily. This number can seem daunting for those trying to establish a regular exercise program, but breaking this target number down into smaller step goals each week and celebrating continual successes can help maintain motivation. There are a number of apps and fitness trackers out there designed to do just that.

Walking throughout the day is preferable to spending most of the day sitting and trying to offset that with a single burst of exercise. All those steps quickly add up, and by spending less time sitting, the brain and body begin to respond more favourably to exercise, meaning that it becomes easier and easier to maintain a healthy walking regimen and regulate appetite.

HOW SITTING INCREASES
THE RISK OF CANCER

It might not seem like the most obvious danger from sitting too much – particularly compared to the well-known threat of cardiovascular disease – but a sedentary lifestyle is increasingly recognised as a major risk factor for more than a dozen types of cancer. In part, this is because too much sitting is directly correlated with weight gain and obesity. However, extended sitting also raises the risk of cancer in lean people.

It's not hyperbole to say that cancer is a disease of modern civilisation. While there are many long-standing natural causes of cancer, and cancer rates have increased in accordance with increases in the average human lifespan, the fact remains that industrialisation and associated lifestyle changes have had a massive impact on the rates of almost all types of cancer.

Societies that maintain a more traditional way of life, involving foraging for food and only occasionally eating animals, have populations that are in many regards healthier than more 'advanced' societies where convenience foods, motorised transport, and sedentary pastimes are the norm. As colonialism spread across the globe, researchers working on the frontiers often noted the relative lack of cancer in native populations compared to rates seen in European societies and, later, in increasingly urbanised populations in America. Colonial science certainly had (and, arguably, has) its problems, but a wealth of evidence from recent research supports the idea that as western civilisation spread around the world, so did cancer.

Modern city living typically means gross reductions in physical activity, as well as changes in diet, and increased exposure to pollution and external stressors. Such lifestyle factors are now well recognised for their role in obesity and diabetes, but few people realise just how much of an impact our urbanised, sedentary lifestyles have on our risk of developing cancer. This list is by no means complete, and new research continues to emerge, but it should illustrate that the danger is very real and backed by solid science.

- Endometrial cancer – two to seven times more likely to develop in overweight or obese women (Setiawan et al., 2013; Dougan et al., 2015)

- Esophageal adenocarcinoma – twice to four times more likely in people who are overweight or obese (Hoyo et al., 2012)

- Gastric cardia cancer – nearly twice as likely in people who are obese (Chen et al., 2013)

- Liver cancer – up to twice as likely in people who are overweight or obese (Chen et al., 2012; Campbell et al., 2016)

- Kidney cancer – nearly twice as likely in those who are overweight (Wang et al., 2014), independent of high blood pressure, which is itself a risk factor for renal cancer (Sanfilippo et al., 2014)

- Multiple myeloma – 10-20% increased risk in people who are overweight or obese (Wallin & Larsson, 2011)

- Meningioma – 20-50% increased risk in people who are overweight or obese (Niedermaier et al., 2015)

- Pancreatic cancer – 150% increased risk in people who are overweight (Genkinger et al., 2011)

- Colorectal cancer – around 30% more likely in those who are obese (Ma et al., 2013)

- Gallbladder cancer – 20-60% increased risk in people who are overweight or obese (World Cancer Research Fund International/American Institute for Cancer Research, 2015; Li et al., 2016)

- Breast cancer – 12% increased risk with every 5-point increase in BMI (Renehan et al., 2008); among postmenopausal women who are obese, the risk is increased by 20-40% (Munsell et al., 2014); obesity also increases the risk for breast cancer in men (Brinton et al., 2014)

- Ovarian cancer – 10% increased risk with every 5-point increase in BMI among women who have never used menopausal hormone therapy (Collaborative Group on Epidemiological Studies of Ovarian

Cancer, 2012)

- Thyroid cancer – 16% increased risk for women and a 21% increased risk for men with every 5-point increase in BMI; regardless of sex, being overweight raised the risk of thyroid cancer by 20%, while being obese raised the risk by 53% (Kitahara et al., 2011)

At this point you might be wondering, what about lean people? Are they off the hook? Science would suggest otherwise.

Even if a person maintains a normal body weight, sedentary behaviour is undeniably associated with underlying biochemical changes that stimulate the development of various cancers.

A sedentary lifestyle reduces the body's ability to respond to insulin, the hormone that helps transport energy in the form of glucose into cells from the blood. In response, the pancreas begins to produce greater amounts of insulin, which is a growth factor for cells, including those which are cancerous (Gallagher et al., 2015).

Researchers have investigated this link by looking specifically at how chronic hyperinsulinemia influences endometrial cancer (Gunter et al, 2008). Hyperinsulinemia, or excess levels of insulin in the blood, appears to directly stimulate the proliferation (growth) of cells that line the uterus (the endometrium). It also contributes indirectly to cancerous growth by increasing levels of insulin-like growth factor-1 (IGF-1) in the endometrium while at the same time decreasing levels of insulin-like growth factor-binding proteins (IGFBP) (Kaaks et al, 2002).

It is also theorised that hyperinsulinemia can increase levels of bioavailable estrogens by decreasing levels of the estrogen-binding protein, sex hormone binding globulin (SHBG) (Kaaks et al, 2002). This is a particular problem for many of the cancers in the aforementioned list, which are hormone-dependent, including endometrial, breast, and ovarian cancer. However, physical activity may help decrease the risk of endometrial cancer, for example, because it reduces blood levels of the hormone estradiol and increases levels of SHBG, the binding protein for estradiol (McTiernan, 2008).

Too much sitting can also trigger a state of constant inflammation, which raises the risk of cancerous modifications (Gregor & Hotamisligil, 2011) and decreases the production of important antioxidant enzymes, such as superoxide dismutase, which leaves the body's cells more vulnerable to damage by free radicals that can cause cancerous mutations (Azizbeigi et al., 2014).

In one meta-analysis, researchers studied almost 70,000 cases of cancer and found that people who were more sedentary had a significantly higher risk of colon, endometrial, and lung cancer. Statistically, for every two hours spent sitting each day, the risk for lung cancer is increased by 6%, colon cancer by 8%, and endometrial cancer by 10%, respectively (Schmid & Leitzmann, 2014). In another study, this time looking at more than 45,000 men, researchers found that, compared with men who mostly sat during work hours, those who sat for half the time had a 20% lower risk of prostate cancer. In fact, every 30 minutes of walking or bicycling lowered the overall risk of prostate cancer by an impressive 12% (Orsini et al., 2009).

The benefits of walking extend far beyond cancer prevention. Research suggests that cancer survivors should avoid prolonged sitting, as this can hamper recovery and make it harder to overcome the deconditioning common amongst those with cancer. Specifically, regular physical activity has been shown to help prevent – or even reverse – the negative effects of cancer and cancer treatment on the heart, muscles, blood vessels, and blood cells (Howden et al., 2018). Walking is an excellent option for those in recovery as it places little physical strain on the body, is easily accessible, low or no monetary cost, and can reduce associated emotional stress.

While we're still just beginning to understand the interconnection between sedentary behaviour and cancer, it seems clear that walking not only helps with weight management, breathing, blood sugar control, and spinal health, but can also dramatically reduce cancer risk, by making our bodies more resilient and better able to recover from disease.

CHAPTER THREE:

HOW SITTING AFFECTS THE MIND

THE BRAIN – MOVE IT OR LOSE IT

The brain is increasingly understood to be more closely related to a muscle than an organ. And, like all muscles, the brain needs movement and exercise to reach and maintain peak performance. In fact, evolutionary science suggests that the very reason humans developed a brain was to enable physical movement. Therefore, by moving less we're effectively regressing to the point of becoming brainless.

Sitting in an office chair every day for hours on end quite literally shrinks the brain. On the other hand, exercise is like fertiliser for brain cells, helping boost your capacity for learning, memory, and problem-solving, while enhancing focus and attention. Exercise helps both mind and body stay limber as you age.

We've all seen spritely nonagenarians (individuals in their nineties) who are sharp as a tack compared to their sedentary peers. Cognitive decline may feel like an inevitable part of ageing, but scientific research now overwhelmingly shows that dementia is irrevocably linked to underactive lifestyles over the decades before we begin to fully lose our faculties. The good news is, exercise offers a significant opportunity to help even older brains reverse degenerative changes and promote learning and growth, thanks to neuroplasticity and neurogenesis.

Sedentary lifestyles are increasingly recognised around the world as being a major contributor to depression, anxiety, dementia, Alzheimer's disease, attention deficit disorder, and numerous other psychiatric conditions. By 2050, more than 130 million people are expected to be living with Alzheimer's disease (Alzheimer's Disease International), which will have far-reaching residual effects on our healthcare system and society as a whole.

A good level of cardiovascular physical fitness during middle-age has been associated with close to a 90% reduction in dementia risk in later life, and is inextricably linked to a host of mental and physical benefits that can be enjoyed for years to come.

So, how exactly is movement such a boon for cognitive health? And what's the best way to exercise to boost brainpower through exercise? Let's dig into the science and see.

WHAT OUR BRAINS ARE ACTUALLY FOR

Descartes famously said, "I think, therefore I am." However, when it comes to matters of the mind, the more apt statement might well be, "I move, therefore I think."

Millions of years ago, most of the creatures on Earth did not have a central nervous system (CNS), let alone anything resembling the human brain. Over thousands of years, the need for movement – specifically adaptable and complex movements to help organisms evade danger and find nourishment – led to the development of the CNS and the brain.

Humans are movers first and foremost, and anthropological research shows that the first regions of the human brain to develop were those areas that control movement. Subsequent brain growth extended outwards from the motor cortex, further adding capacity that allowed us to better think, plan and predict. Thinking is the evolutionary internalisation of movement as the nerve cells that are stimulated when we move are the same as those needed for other, higher order cognitive functions. Put simply, if we weren't movers, we wouldn't be thinkers.

As recently as 10,000 years ago, we were hunter-gatherers covering somewhere between 10-14 miles a day. Now, most of us spend around 12 hours a day sitting and staring at screens. And we wonder why it is so hard to concentrate! Our brains are suffering because our behaviour is essentially sending the signal that we don't need all that gray matter after all.

This idea is supported by research courtesy of the Semel Institute for

Neuroscience and Human Behavior at the University of California Los Angeles (UCLA). Through magnetic resonance imaging (MRI), researchers were able to investigate the effects of sedentary behaviour on the brain in middle-aged and older adults currently living without dementia. The volunteers also underwent cognitive testing and were asked about their levels of physical activity and the average number of hours each day they spent sitting. The researchers found that the more hours people spent sitting each day, the thinner the tissue in their medial temporal lobe (MTL). This region of the brain includes an area called the hippocampus, which is largely responsible for storing and accessing memory. Essentially, prolonged periods of sitting during middle age can adversely affect the physical construction of the brain, which in turn negatively impacts our ability to process information. Sit for too long and the MTL becomes thin, even in people who try to offset sedentary behaviour with regular exercise. Conversely, physical movement enhances the thickness of the MTL and actively protects against memory loss and cognitive decline in older age, as well as results in improved cognitive performance at every stage of life (Siddarth et al., 2018).

One of the key findings in this study is that it's not simply a lack of physical activity that raises the risk of early onset dementia and cognitive decline. Rather, sedentary behaviour is an *independent risk factor* for brain atrophy. Many people who are highly active – heading to the gym before or after work – are still sedentary for most of their day. This important detail helps explain why researchers may struggle to identify specific benefits of exercise interventions for cognitive health and emotional wellbeing. It's not exercise alone that boosts brain health; it's overall fitness and avoidance of an inactive lifestyle.

Why do movement and fitness matter so much when it comes to maintaining a healthy brain? Part of the answer lies within a range of chemicals including neurotransmitters and something called brain-derived neurotrophic factor (BDNF).

BDNF – THE BRAIN FERTILISER

In the 1990s neuroscience underwent a rapid period of discovery, uncovering exciting insights into how the brain can actually incite growth. Thanks to technology such as MRI and spectroscopy, as well as chemicals able to bind to BDNF, researchers could see for the first time that stem cells in the brain were forming new neurons (neurogenesis). This was remarkable, particularly given that the understanding within the scientific community up to this point was that, once a person lost brain cells after damage from a stroke, for instance, the skills and functions associated with that area of brain tissue had also been lost for good.

It was also widely accepted that brain development stops after childhood, and that, as adults we have to work with the finite gray matter we have and face inevitable atrophy and loss of brain cells as we age. We now know that stem cells stick around for our whole lives, allowing for the development of new brain cells and connections, thanks to biomechanisms involving brain-derived neurotrophic factor (BDNF), other neurotransmitters, and the right external stimuli. This effect is known as neuroplasticity – basically the potential to keep developing new neural pathways in response to our physical environment, including exercise – and neurogenesis – the process of growing new brain cells.

These revelations about the brain were industry game changers. If the brain could grow new cells and form new connections regardless of a person's age or circumstances, there was significant hope for our ability to rewire the brain after injury and perhaps even reverse or prevent cognitive decline and dysfunction over time.

Further research found that, while lifelong learning boosts neuroplasticity and neurogenesis, nothing enhances these processes like living an active lifestyle with lots of movement throughout the day. Put simply, just as exercise is key to muscle growth, it is also vital for helping the brain grow stronger, more resilient, and more flexible. In the human brain, thousands of new neurons are added every day; unfortunately, most of these new cells don't survive long, with more than half dying within weeks of development (Shors et al., 2012). The trick to keeping these neurons alive and well is to stimulate the cells through ongoing learning combined with a diverse set of physical activity.

Physical movement increases the number of stem cells in our brain tissue, creating a larger pool of new neurons (Blackmore et al., 2009). So, even if most new neurons continue to die shortly after being created, those who stay active have a higher number to start with and a higher number left over. And, by combining consistent exercise with intellectual activity, we retain more of these brain cells and enhance our overall brain capacity. This two-step process shows that it takes both continual exercise and a commitment to learning in order to become smarter. We'll come back to this, but first let's look more closely at the neurotrophic factors, including BDNF, that help spark neurogenesis and facilitate lifelong learning.

EXERCISE AND BDNF

Brain-derived neurotrophic factor (BDNF) was first discovered in 1989 by Yves-Alain Barde and Hans Thoenen while studying the brain tissue of pigs. BDNF is a neurotrophin, as well as a nerve growth factor (NGF), neurotrophin 3 (NT3), and neurotrophin 4 (NT4). Its most important functions include neuronal developmental, regulation of synaptogenesis, neuroprotection, and control of synapse activity influencing memory and cognition (Kowiański et al., 2018).

The brain releases BDNF in response to the increased mental demands associated with movement, which triggers brain cell growth and further release of BDNF. As BDNF floods the brain, it fundamentally changes the structure and function of brain tissue, making it easier to learn, consolidate information and skills, and to stay sharp, active, and motivated both physically and mentally. BDNF is at once both the fertiliser and the landscaper of the brain.

At the time of writing, there are over 1,300 published papers looking at the relationship between BDNF and exercise, including at least 50 clinical trials investigating the effects of physical activity on BDNF in human volunteers.

In a 2010 review of randomised controlled trials, Smith and colleagues looked at the effects of aerobic exercise on neurocognitive performance. They included 29 studies, involving over 2,000 volunteers, and conclusively found that exercise was associated with improvements in attention and processing speed, as well as executive function and memory. One study found that high impact, short exertion anaerobic running led to significant increases in BDNF and catecholamine (epinephrine, dopamine and

64

norepinephrine) levels and enabled volunteers to learn new vocabulary 20% faster than volunteers who rested. (Winter et al., 2007). The results also showed that more sustained BDNF levels during learning following intense exercise seemed to facilitate better short-term learning, while dopamine was linked to improved immediate retention of new vocabulary, and epinephrine to our long-term memory.

Several studies looking at the neuroprotective effects of BDNF have involved people with multiple sclerosis (MS), a disease that leads to progressive loss of the insulating sheath around the nerves. In one study, BDNF levels were found to be 21% lower in people with MS, compared to healthy controls. After a 24-week exercise intervention, BDNF levels in the MS patients increased by an average of roughly 15%, whereas volunteers assigned to a sedentary control group had decreases in BDNF of around 10%. The exercise group, but not the sedentary group, also saw improvements in muscle strength, exercise tolerance, and body composition (Wens et al., 2016). A review of studies examining the effects of aerobic exercise on BDNF levels in people with neurodegenerative disorders like MS found that, while a large effect was seen with a regular exercise program, even a single bout of exercise had minimal effect, strongly suggesting that daily walking can be incredibly advantageous for people living with neurological disorders (Mackay et al., 2017).

The stark reality is that sedentary behaviour has fast and direct negative effects on neurogenesis, brain plasticity, neurotrophin (BDNF) production, angiogenesis, and control of inflammation and pathological processes that contribute to cognitive decline, anxiety, depression, and even neurodegenerative disease (Chastin et al., 2014).

HOW SEDENTARY BEHAVIOUR
AFFECTS OUR ABILITY TO LEARN

The importance of movement in learning is now recognised by many health and education authorities worldwide. Among them includes the United States National Institute of Medicine, which recommends that fitness-based physical education should be a core school subject, not because of physical health, but because of its direct benefits for learning. In one school district, teachers took these early neuroscience findings to heart and implemented a fitness-based learning model that has had startling benefits.

In the Naperville school district in Illinois, students engage in a minimum of 40 minutes of active movement each day while at school. This doesn't mean standing around idly on a football field or waiting for a pass on the basketball court. Instead, students take part in activities designed to get their heart rate up to 75-80% of their maximum, whatever that figure may be. The kids run, perform calisthenics, climb, dance, and participate in other pursuits every day. What's more, guidance counsellors have begun to schedule the kids' hardest subjects immediately following fitness classes so as to maximise their post-workout learning potential.

To back this up with data, in a country where a third of children were overweight in 2003, just 3% of Naperville kids were overweight the year after the implementation of this new system (Ratey, 2008). And, in the Trends in International Mathematics and Science Study (TIMSS) used to assess students' knowledge across countries, Naperville kids (who competed as a country themselves) came in first in the world for science and sixth in the world for mathematics (Ratey, 2008). For comparison, the U.S. as a whole came in eighteenth and nineteenth in science and mathematics, respectively.

Seeing the success following the Naperville system, researchers have scrambled to determine the underlying factors that drive these positive changes in overall health and academic performance. Subsequent research, including the FITkids study, has found that daily exercise has significant benefits for executive control, accuracy, and reaction times in kids as young as seven (Hillman et al., 2014). Other studies have found that physical activity improves oxygen delivery to the brain, which in turn enhances bone and muscle strength in kids, and increases resistance to stress (Frischenschlager & Gosch, 2012).

Conversely, sedentary kids who engage more frequently in passive activities, such as watching TV or playing seated video games, have more difficulty with attention, focus, and behavioural issues compared to their active peers who demonstrate better reaction times and visual selective attention (Alesi et al., 2014; Syväoja et al., 2014). These studies, and others like them, overwhelmingly support a positive effect of physical fitness on academic achievement in school children (Castelli et al., 2007; Chomitz et al., 2009).

While studies about learning are most often applied to children or adolescents, there's plenty of evidence supporting the cognitive usefulness of regular physical activity in adults, as well as the perils of too little.

In one study with older adults, a six-month program of daily brisk walking not only led to significant improvements in cardiorespiratory fitness, but also to improved executive function, including reasoning, working memory, and task-switching abilities (Baniqued et al., 2018).

The research investigating the relationship between physical fitness and cognitive function becomes a little more complex in adulthood, in part because adults tend to be better at compensating for reduced capacity in some cognitive tasks by calling on other skills (Kamijo et al., 2010). In addition, research suggests that it is not high intensity aerobic fitness that predicts cognitive health. Rather, an active versus a sedentary lifestyle seems to be a better predictor of robust cognitive function throughout the lifespan.

In one study, researchers found that higher levels of physical activity at the age of 36 was associated with a significantly slower rate of memory decline from ages 43-53, with further protective effects when physical activity continued during that time (Richards et al., 2003). In a large study involving 2,509 older adults, those who were more physically active were 31% more likely to maintain cognitive function over the following eight years compared to their more sedentary peers (Yaffe et al., 2009).

Just as it's essential to build and maintain strong, healthy bones through load-bearing exercise, it's also vital to exercise the brain to build new tissue and create new connections. The better one's brain function at midlife, the more likely a person is to maintain cognitive health into his or her golden years. That said, even in cases where cognitive decline has become apparent, exercise has continually proven to help decelerate – and even reverse – cognitive impairment in older age.

SEDENTARY BEHAVIOUR
AND THE RISK OF DEMENTIA

Every three seconds someone in the world develops dementia. A staggering 50 million people are currently thought to be living with dementia, a number that is expected to rise to an unprecedented 131.5 million by 2050. The global cost of dementia is estimated at more than a trillion U.S. dollars, including direct medical costs and the costs of informal and social care (Alzheimer's Disease International). These figures do not take into account the cost associated with lost productivity, with the assumption that older adults are no longer in the workforce.

In many countries, retirement age has increased dramatically, meaning that dementia is ever more likely to strike while individuals are continuing to work for an income.

Most people now know that avoiding smoking, maintaining a healthy body weight, and staying intellectually and socially stimulated can help to stave off dementia. However, daily Sudokus will make little difference when an individual spends most of his or her day sitting.

A longitudinal study that followed the health of women for up to 44 years recently found that those with a high level of cardiovascular fitness in middle-age had an 88% reduced risk of dementia in later life compared to those who were only considered moderately fit. Up to 23% of the women in this study developed dementia over the 44-year period, but the highly-fit women who developed dementia did so an average of eleven years later than their sedentary peers (at 90 vs. 79 years old). After adjusting for body weight, the women with the lowest levels of fitness at age 44 had a significantly higher risk of dementia compared to women with medium fitness levels. Just 5% of the women in the highly-fit group developed dementia, compared to 25% of the medium-fitness group, 32% of the low-fitness group and a staggering 45% of those who were unable to finish the fitness test at age 44, respectively (Hörder et al., 2018).

Another analysis, looking at results from several studies concerned with the influence of fitness on dementia, came to a similar result. Adults over the age of 65 who were physically active had a 39% reduced risk of developing Alzheimer's disease when compared to their non-active peers (Beckett et al., 2015).

One study of particular interest within the context of this book, looked at the hours spent sitting each day against the risk of poor mental health in later life. Compared to those who did not engage in leisure-time physical activity, active older adults had improved scores on emotional and mental wellbeing, as well as physical and social functioning, lowered bodily pain and heightened vitality. As found in many comparable studies, the number of hours spent sitting were inversely related with most of the scores used to assess quality of life (Balboa-Castillo et al., 2011).

The good news is that – just as you can always sabotage your health by sitting too much – it's never too late to reap the benefits of exercise for one's cognitive health. In fact, evidence strongly suggests that, even if an individual has poor fitness at age 44, switching sedentary behaviour for an active lifestyle can result in cognitive benefits later in life and a more healthy ageing process.

The benefits of exercise in preventing against Alzheimer's disease (and dementia in general) shouldn't be all that surprising given that the condition is associated with an excessive loss of neurons, particularly in the hippocampus and cerebral cortex. In autopsies of the parietal cortex of people with Alzheimer's disease, researchers found a 3.4-fold decrease in the levels of BDNF microRNA, compared to controls without the condition (Holsinger et al., 2000). This decrease of BDNF in brain tissue is not only likely to contribute to dementia, but may also come as a result of dementia, given that people with Alzheimer's disease are often more sedentary (both voluntarily and due to care practices) than their more active peers.

Maintaining physical activity and fitness in later life has also been found to help with emotional wellbeing. In one study, older adults who spent more time engaged in light physical activity, such as walking, scored higher on an Alzheimer's quality of life test, which included better muscle strength and a significantly lower risk of depression (Arrieta et al., 2018).

MOVEMENT OVER MEDICATION
FOR MENTAL HEALTH

The message is clear: people who are sedentary are almost twice as likely to be depressed as those who are physically active. According to a recent analysis of data from over 40,000 people, individuals under the age of 65 who sat for eight or more hours a day had a 94% increased risk of being depressed (Stubbs et al., 2018). With statistics such as these, it is hard to deny that we have a considerable amount of control when it comes to our mental and emotional state.

How is sitting linked to common mental health issues, such as depression and anxiety? Depression is now viewed by many physicians as being a consequence of the brain, i.e. through the loss of functional capacity as a result of decreased neurons and decelerated activity at the synapses. One recent study found that ceasing regular exercise directly increased depressive symptoms in healthy adults, particularly amongst women (Morgan et al., 2018).

Research linking exercise to improved mental health is nothing new. Studies began to investigate this idea back in the late 1970s, with significant work carried out at Duke University. As part of a long history of cardiac rehabilitation studies, researchers looked at the effects of A) exercise (in the form of treadmill walking or jogging) as treatment for people with depression and coronary heart disease, comparing it to B) treatment in the form of a placebo, C) treatment with the antidepressant sertraline (Zoloft), and D) a combination of Zoloft and exercise. After 16 weeks, exercise and Zoloft were found to be equally effective in reducing depressive symptoms, with a significantly greater effect compared to placebo treatment. Exercise had the added benefit of improving a measure of heart function (Blumenthal et al., 2012).

Early research found that patients who engaged in a walking program for cardiac rehabilitation tended to become less stressed, less aggressive, and happier, as well as more physically fit. In one early study in this field, Blumenthal and colleagues recruited healthy middle-aged volunteers and assessed the effects of continued sedentary behaviour versus a ten-week walking/jogging program on mental health. They found that almost everyone in the exercise group had improvements in their respective anxiety levels, decreased tension, depression, and fatigue, and more vigor than those who remained sedentary (Blumenthal et al., 1982).

Walking has also demonstrated a range of mood benefits in people living with a variety of chronic diseases and conditions. In a study of individuals being treated with chemotherapy for breast cancer, a 12-week, home-based, self-paced walking program was seen to have improvements in fatigue, mood, and self-esteem (Gokal et al., 2016). A similar program was associated with improvements in perceived stress and depression symptoms in people who had suffered a traumatic brain injury (TBI) (Bellon et al., 2015).

There's no shortage of studies that exalt the benefits of walking to suppress depression. One study found that, in postmenopausal women with depression, a six-month moderate intensity walking intervention (three times a week, 40 minutes per session) led to significant improvements in depression compared to a control group assigned to a wait list (Bernard et al., 2015).

Given all we know about the benefits of exercise for the brain, the idea that movement can also benefit our psychological health isn't all that surprising. The same mechanisms that support cognitive functioning also support emotional functioning; this includes improved dopamine receptivity and activity, neurogenesis and neuroplasticity, and better all-round metabolism in brain tissue due to improved circulation and nutrient uptake (Schoenfeld & Cameron, 2015).

BDNF plays a major role in brain function and has been implicated in the pathology of depression. People with depression are consistently found to have low levels of BDNF; given this known connection, it should come as no surprise that researchers have sought to harness its power and use BDNF within antidepressants. (Polyakova et al., 2015). So far, however, this has yet to be achieved in any meaningful way.

Between the brain and body is an effective feedback loop, whereby we create more BDNF when we use brain cells. And, as we already know, nothing increases BDNF like exercise, not even meditation or learning. We use more brain cells during physical activity than any other, leading to a flood of BDNF that promotes neuroplasticity, and dopamine and serotonin activity.

Improving neuroplasticity may, in theory, be particularly helpful for those who experience a certain kind of circular thinking typically seen in depression and other mental ailments. By enhancing the brain's ability to form new connections and to effectively rewire itself, people may be better able to break free from their well-trodden negative thought patterns. This idea was borne out of research showing that exercise improves the response to cognitive behavioural therapy and medication in the treatment of depression (Gourgouvelis et al., 2018). Astonishingly, in one small study, an eight-week exercise intervention led to a therapeutic response (or, in some, complete remission) of depression symptoms in 75% of patients, compared to just 25% of those engaging solely in cognitive behavioural therapy with medication. Exercise also improved the participants' sleep quality and cognitive function, and increased their BDNF levels in tandem with decreased symptoms of depression. With research upon research demonstrating similar findings, it's surprising that physical exercise isn't seen more often as part of the 'doctor's orders.'

Recent research in mice has found that BDNF levels correspond with novelty-seeking exploratory behaviour, suggesting that BDNF not only supports motivation but may also act as a comfort during new experiences. Indeed, administering BDNF to mice with an avoidant or balanced disposition was shown to increase exploratory behaviour (Laricchiuta et al., 2018). This may mean that by engaging in regular exercise and avoiding sedentary behaviour, humans who typically feel anxious in new situations may begin to feel more adventurous and comfortable with novel experiences.

Put simply, BDNF manipulation through the avoidance of sedentary behaviour offers significant opportunity for individuals to overcome their reluctance to exercise, and provides benefits for the mind, body, and overall health and happiness. In study after study, researchers have confirmed the benefits of movement – especially walking – for managing anxiety, depression, attention deficit disorder, obsessive-compulsive disorder, and even addictions, schizophrenia, and bipolar disorder. In many ways, movement is more effective than medication for treating and preventing mental health problems, and with far less consequences! In 2010, the American Psychiatric Association recognised for the first time that exercise is a proven treatment for depression.

Medications and psychotherapy can be expensive, inaccessible, have side effects, and be of limited use for many individuals. Not to mention the stigma that continues to surround mental health in many communities. Considering how depression and other mental health issues often have an underlying metabolic component, it makes intuitive sense to prescribe physical activity to combat depression and support ongoing mental health.

GIVE UP YOUR CHAIR
TO BETTER MANAGE STRESS

How can exercise help improve our ability to resist the negative effects of stress? Part of the answer is through neurogenesis, specifically new growth of neurons and reorganisation of neurons mediated by the inhibitory neurotransmitter gamma amino butyric acid (GABA). This neurotransmitter has the ability to constrain excitatory neurotransmitter activity and slow our innate fight or flight response (Ma, 2008; Sah et al., 2017). In animal studies, rats who spent more time engaged in physical activity had higher GABA levels in key brain areas and were less vulnerable to the effects of stress (Molteni et al., 2002). Put simply, the fitter you are, the more stress you can effectively manage. When stress is particularly high, it activates the sympathetic nervous system, affecting the hippocampus, which is both the memory centre and the area of the brain that predominantly controls anxiety and panic.

There's a reason why hot-headed people are told to 'take a walk' to cool off. An acute bout of exercise is like taking a bit of both Prozac and Ritalin; it effectively calms anxiety levels and cheers us up while allowing us to direct our focus to the situation at hand. Exercise increases norepinephrine, serotonin, and dopamine, which modulate the entire range of neurorunctional systems such as attention, aggression, motivation, concentration, alertness, memory, anxiety, irritability, mood, reward, and pleasure. And, of course, exercise increases BDNF, the brain's fertiliser.

Most people have heard of a 'runner's high,' usually attributed to endorphins released during exercise. What many people don't realise, however, is that we also create our own marijuana-like neurohormones, called endocannabinoids, which are released when we experience injury. These endocannabinoids effectively calm the brain and help us feel happy and comforted. In tests with mice, endocannabinoids increased with voluntary physical activity (such as running) and have been associated with decreased anxiety, pain sensitivity, and sedation, effectively recreating a runner's high in the animals; mice given a substance that blocks the effects of endocannabinoids did not experience these positive effects with exercise (Fuss et al., 2015).

'MENS SANA IN CORPORE SANO' – A HEALTHY MIND IN A HEALTHY BODY

We have covered a lot in this chapter, spanning from the evolution of the human brain, to how exercise can be an effective treatment for depression and anxiety. We have explored the vast cerebral risks associated with sedentary life – which can literally shrink the brain – and shown how staying active throughout one's life can dramatically reduce the risk of cognitive decline.

In the final part of this chapter, we offer support for the idea that cognitive health cannot be fully understood solely by studying the brain, but rather should incorporate the complex connections between mind and body, such as the gut-brain axis. What's more, these connections do not stop with our own organs, tissues, and cells: a wealth of evidence now shows that the microbiome (the bacteria and other organisms within the body) interacts with our own cells to add yet another dimension to our health and wellbeing.

FROM THE BRAIN TO THE BODY AND BACK

Humans have twelve pairs of nerves that originate in the brain and extend throughout the body. One of these, the vagus nerve, connects the brain to various organs and is an integral part of the parasympathetic nervous system. Often referred to as the 'rest and digest' nerve, the vagus is involved in feelings of relaxation, comfort, tranquility, and diminished anxiety and stress. It is this system that allows us to maintain our equilibrium during times of stress; when it becomes maladaptive and inflexible, somatic and psychological effects can result.

On its journey down to the gut, the vagus nerve oversees a vast array of vital processes in the body, including immune response, digestion, and heart rate. Staying within the realm of physical activity and health, we will focus on the vagal modulation of the heart and gut. Since measuring vagal tone is mostly done by using a parameter called Heart Rate Variability (HRV), let's briefly look the theory behind this metric and explore how to interpret HRV correctly.

HEART RATE VARIABILITY

Measuring stress is a highly subjective endeavor. There is no single way to conclusively and uniformly determine degrees of stress, and although measuring levels of certain stress hormones, such as cortisol, in the blood can prove useful in controlled clinical studies, such measurements are simply not practical in everyday life, as they are influenced by a number of other factors, such as the circadian rhythm and environmental stimuli.

Another widely used physiological parameter, heart rate variability (HRV), is significantly more practical and accessible. And, thanks to improvements in accuracy and the increased availability of consumer devices, this decades-old measurement has become something of a proxy for physical and mental health today.

But what exactly is HRV? And how can it help us measure stress and resilience? Let's start by refuting the widely held belief that the heart beats at a constant frequency. This is simply not the case. A healthy heart within a healthy individual will adapt its rhythm to match the needs of a given situation. Even in a resting state, there are micro adjustments between two single heart beats. Once detected, these tiny differences can provide a measurement of the variability of one's heart rate. If the intervals between heartbeats are near constant, the HRV is low. By the same token, if the interval between beats changes with greater frequency, the HRV is high.

HRV has become a popular way for individuals to track training status, offering insights that can alert a person to problems (such as overtraining), as well as indicate overall adaptation and fitness. In the context of this chapter, heart rate variability is inextricably linked to the autonomic nervous system and the vagus nerve, with a higher vagal tone resulting in a lower heart rate and a higher HRV. In stressful situations that trigger our fight or flight response, the parasympathetic nervous system becomes subdued and is replaced by activity in the sympathetic branch, facilitating an increase in heart rate and lower HRV.

As there are various methods for calculating HRV, and since HRV values differ from person to person, there is no definitive consensus over an ideal HRV value. That said, the most robust data is typically collected using nighttime measurements where tracking conditions remain largely constant, thereby minimising possible confounding variables.

VAGAL TONE IN HEALTH AND DISEASE

An increasing body of evidence shows that regular engagement in physical activity can help modulate vagal tone with measurable effects on HRV. In one study, researchers found that regular exercise in young healthy men led to improved vagal tone that was apparently associated with increased hippocampal connectivity; the men's brains changed in response to exercise, and was linked to a greater ability to regulate heart rate (Bär et al., 2016).

Studies show that even a single bout of high intensity exercise can positively influence vagal signaling (Guiraud et al., 2013). However, the greatest benefits for vagal tone come from consistent physical activity and reduced sedentary behaviour, as well as deep diaphragmatic breathing that is associated with better posture and relaxing meditative exercises (Servant et al., 2009).

It's easy to see how reduced physical activity and a hunched posture while sitting can have overwhelmingly negative effects on vagal tone and overall psychological health. People suffering from depression and anxiety disorders have been shown to have abnormal HRV compared to peers without mental health issues (Servant et al., 2009). Generally, it can be assumed that the vagal tone is linked to our ability to regulate emotions, with poorer tone associated with greater social anxiety, defensiveness, impaired attention, and maladaptive avoidance responses (Aldao et al., 2016; Movius & Allen, 2005).

THE MICROBIOME AND THE MIND – TYING IT ALL TOGETHER

When most people think about matters of the mind, they think of the brain, not the gut. In recent years, however, the science has stacked up dramatically to support the importance of the gut-brain axis on our overall psychological and physical wellbeing. As such, we can't talk about the sedentary mind without discussing the impact of physical activity (or inactivity) on the microbiome, and how the gut itself can influence our desire and capacity for movement. It should also be noted that the gut-brain axis is bi-directional, meaning that what happens in the brain also affects the gut in an ongoing feedback loop.

One of the major factors affecting gut health and, therefore, brain health, is the makeup of our microbiome, i.e. the diversity of bacteria and other microorganisms in our gastrointestinal tract, skin, airways, and genitourinary tract. These microorganisms outnumber our own cells and play a significant role in virtually all aspects of our health. They synthesise nutrients, create compounds that regulate inflammation and immune function, influence gene expression, help break down toxins and, in the case of pathogens, produce toxins. These microorganisms can even synthesise neurotransmitters that affect our mood, desires, sensitivity to pain, and our ability to think clearly.

On the other side of the coin, our emotional state also affects our microbiome. If we feel stressed, depressed, anxious, or relaxed, this can change the conditions in our gastrointestinal tract, which in turn affects the microorganisms that live there.

Our understanding of the microbiome and its effects on psychological and cognitive health has increased substantially and rapidly in recent years. Research has found, for instance, that people who are sedentary have a significantly less diverse and robust microbiome when compared to more active people. This predisposes those who are less active to a greater risk of immune system dysfunction, poor digestion, allergies and intolerances, undesirable inflammation, bowel disease, and a host of negative cognitive and psychological consequences (Barton et al., 2018).

Fortunately, sedentary people can bolster the health of their microbiome by increasing their level of physical activity (Cronin et al., 2018), which also serves to decrease chronic low-level inflammation. This persistent inflammation has been increasingly recognised as a cornerstone of most chronic non-infectious diseases (Clarke et al., 2014), suggesting that modifying the microbiome could have major consequences for lifelong health and happiness. Indeed, many of the health benefits associated with being physically active are, at least in part, mediated by the microbiome and microbe-host interactions. These include prevention and treatment of age-related cognitive impairment, prevention of various types of cancer, diabetes, and cardiovascular disease, prevention and management of irritable bowel syndrome, and psychological disorders including depression, anxiety, and obsessive-compulsive disorder (O'Sullivan et al., 2015).

No single organ or system in the body can be understood in isolation. Our latest example, the vagus nerve and the microbiome, form a microbe-gut-brain axis, which has far-reaching effects on neurotransmitters, neurohormones, and the hypothalamic-pituitary axis (our central stress response system). As such, the makeup of our microbiome, as influenced by our choice to be sedentary or active, seems to exert profound effects on the regulation of our mood, appetite, digestion, and even sleep and motivation (O'Sullivan et al., 2015). It is paramount that we – as individuals as well as society as a whole – understand this internal interconnection as a remarkable opportunity to tap into a sophisticated and comprehensive feedback system, where increased physical activity helps to increase motivation, leading to better overall cognition and emotional health.

CHAPTER FOUR:
A SCIENTIFIC TAKE ON POSSIBLE SOLUTIONS

EXERCISE IS NOT ENOUGH –
MEET THE ACTIVE COUCH POTATO

The World Health Organization recommends 150 minutes of moderately intensive aerobic exercise per week. Most national health institutions advise a level of exercise within this same range. The fundamental question remains: does this recommendation stand up to the claim that this amount of physical exercise is sufficient for maintaining one's physical and mental health? If you do the math, 150 minutes per week equates to a bit more than 20 minutes of exercise per day. Could such a short time frame be sufficient to counterweight the health hazards associating with sitting for 12 hours or more a day? Recent evidence overwhelmingly suggests that this is not the case, and that even a more intense daily exercise regimen can simply not undo the unfavourable metabolic impact that results from being sedentary for the vast remainder of our waking hours.

First off, do we really sit that much? You may be surprised to read these figures, but the time quickly adds up. The average office employee sits for around two-thirds of their work day, and those who sit the most at work also appear to sit more during transit, after work, and during weekends (Clemes et al., 2014). A French study involving 35,444 working adults with a mean age of 44.5, found similar patterns of behaviour. Working adults sat for an average of 12.15 hours on any given workday, and the more often they sat at work, the more likely they were to be sedentary outside of work (Saidj et al., 2015).

Let's consider the individual who does tend to sit a lot, but also regularly finds time for exercise. The term 'active coach potato' may not sound too charming, but it effectively sums up the lifestyle of the vast majority of those with office jobs. With so much time spent being sedentary in an office environment, you would think that people would be anxious to fill their leisure time with exercise and movement. However, the unfortunate reality is that sitting tends to yield more sitting. We live in a world with increasing professional demands, with many jobs demanding 50 hours or more of our time and attention each week. Not to mention the host of responsibilities and engagements most of us have outside of the office. This can make the idea of engaging in daily exercise seem like an unattainable illusion for many.

Let's shed some further light on this topic. First off, we must determine whether exercise can counter the risks of a sedentary lifestyle, or rather, if extended periods of sitting constitute an independent risk factor, regardless of activity level. A recent scientific study, published in the 2013 Annals of Internal Medicine, investigated this very question (Biswas et al., 2015). The authors conducted an impressive meta-analysis, distilling 47 previously performed studies, looking at all-cause mortality, cardiovascular disease mortality, cardiovascular disease incidence, cancer mortality, cancer incidence, and type 2 diabetes incidence in adults with the above described lifestyle (mainly passive, with short amounts of regular exercise). The conclusion was that prolonged sedentary time is *independently associated* with health risks, regardless of the amount of time an individual spends engaged in physical activity.

The results of this study constituted a paradigm shift within the scientific community which, with the help of supporting research, spread beyond academic circles and led to the rise of the popular headline comparing the risks of sitting with those of smoking. The comparison is a good one. If you are a smoker, you are still at risk to be diagnosed with lung cancer despite also being an active runner. By the same principle, if you maintain a sedentary lifestyle, there is still the same level of threat for heart disease, cancer, diabetes, overweight, dementia and many other chronic diseases, regardless of engaging in regular physical activity. Exercise cannot counter the negative effects of these dangerous habits. When evaluating one's health, sitting time must be considered independently from time spent being active. With the exception of elite athletes who train vigorously for over 60-75 minutes at a time, the time you spend sitting each day cannot be reversed (Ekelund et al., 2017).

Let's back that up with some more data. Activity patterns of more than 220,000 Australians 45 years and older were analysed in a 2012 study, published in Archives of Internal Medicine. The scientists linked prospective questionnaire data from people living in New South Wales and compared daily sitting time with all causes of mortality in that population. Measures were taken to ensure that variables such as sex, age, education, place of living, and smoking status did not falsify the data. The study concluded, once again, that the more hours spent sitting, the greater the chance of dying prematurely. Furthermore, research indicated that an individual's risk didn't change even if part of the day was spent exercising (Van der Ploeg et al., 2012).

While this has been proven repeatedly across a number of scientific studies, the reality has yet to enter the public awareness and therefore affect how we shape our professional and educational spaces. The widespread belief is that going for an evening run a couple of times per week puts you off the hook. If it were only so simple!

In attempt to provide a better understanding and identify possible ways to alleviate this risk, we must consider the human body from both a macroscopic as well as a molecular level. Observations from the field of evolutionary biology hint where we can expect to find possible solutions. Our nomadic ancestors walked for most of the day and even our agrarian ancestors likely only sat for around three hours a day. When comparing against the grand scale of human existence on Earth, it is only in the past 150 years or so in which sedentariness rapidly became the unquestioned status quo. This period of time feels insignificant when considering the big picture in which the human genetic setup developed. Nevertheless, each cell in our body still contains the very same genetic code as our ancestors, which has prepared us for an entirely different status quo: that of an active mover.

Let's dig into this a bit further. When we sit for a long time, muscle contractions – particularly in the legs – largely cease. The problem with this, contrary to popular belief, is not that our muscles are overall losing strength, but rather that the muscle contractions are not able to effectively serve their lesser known, second vital function. Our muscles are responsible for far more than moving a bone or a limb from position A to position B; in fact, they are an integral part of our whole cardiovascular system which, consisting of our heart and blood vessels, is in charge of transporting blood throughout our arteriovenous system. When our muscles don't contract, immediately two things happen: first, they require less blood sugar to operate, and second, as pointed out above, blood begins to collect in the legs due to the force of gravity.

These two seemingly simple physical and physiological principles have huge implications which, in the same metabolic pathway, can end up increasing the effects of one another. Let's consider this in greater detail.

With the muscular pump effectively being switched off, less blood makes its way through our body, including to the brain. The brain has a steady and permanent demand for energy in form of glucose, which is essential to ensuring that our body continues to function properly. As a consequence, our ancestral brain will always interpret reduced leg movement as a highly unnatural state, probably the result of an injury, such as an animal attack. In order to give us the best chance for survival in such a situation, the brain signals the body to increase the level of blood sugar and decrease the level of fat burning. As we discussed earlier, the brain enforces its survival needs through the release of hormones and gene regulation, all in favour of a single goal: to deliver energy to the brain in form of glucose as fast as possible. What had once been a basic physiological survival mechanism has

89

now become a metabolic liability.

However, the problem of increased blood sugar is not solely caused by the top-down demands of the brain; it also results from a bottom-up principle of when the muscles are not moving. When not in need, our musculature naturally requires less energy. This results in a surplus of free fatty acids, which slows fat burning and creates an overall metabolic state that will only become more inflexible over the years. This will undoubtedly have far reaching effects and may set the stage for more 'societal-based diseases.'

It is clear that simply no amount of exercise or level of fitness can change our body's natural response in the described scenarios. Regardless of who we are, we have all been wired in the same way; each of our brains will interpret prolonged sitting simply as inactivity of large muscle groups combined with an unnatural posture. While serious athletes do have a different basic metabolic rate (BMR), meaning that, even when resting, the muscles that have been conditioned to be in regular heavy use will handle caloric intake in a different way than a less active individual. However, even this difference doesn't cut the edge and still renders highly trained individuals almost as likely to be affected by the health hazards of sitting as untrained individuals.

Furthermore, the effect of exercise on overall energy expenditure and impact of net daily sitting time has likely been overestimated. In Finland, a nation well-known for their wearable tracking devices, researchers employed a study in which active participants wore shorts designed with electrodes to measure the electric activity in the large leg muscles. The participants wore these trackers continuously over a number of days, regardless of whether they engaged in exercise or not. The study revealed two interesting facts. First, the amount of time spent exercising had no effect on the time spent in a sedentary posture for the remainder of the day. And second, the increase in energy expenditure on workout days was relatively small, averaging only 13% of the median increase on exercise days. It is clear that such a low margin would not suffice to have an impact large enough to influence the overall metabolism of one's body.

Having such data available demonstrates that even daily exercise simply cannot result in a change profound enough to alter the basic way that humans breakdown nutrients, such as triglycerides. This very question was addressed in a study at the University of Texas at Austin. The participants resembled the classic active couch potato lifestyle. The healthy young men took part in three five-day trials. In the first trial, the men sat for more than 14 hours per day and took in more calories than they were able to burn. The second five-day period took place after a waiting period of more than week, in order to minimise any potential residual effects. In this trial, the men also had to spend over 14 hours of their days being sedentary, but their calorie intake matched the energy they were burning. In the final five-day trail, the men had to walk for around 17,000 steps per day, but spent the rest of the day in a sedentary posture. In each of the three different trial settings, the participants ate a high-fat breakfast on the third and fifth morning, respectively. Also on these days, the subjects ran on a treadmill for one hour with high intensity.

The aim of the study was to look how each pattern of sitting influenced the way the body handles a fatty meal by measuring the free fatty acids floating in the blood after consuming a high-caloric breakfast. The main takeaway was that the body handles fat intake irrespective of exercise, and that prolonged sitting for 2-4 days in a row can lead to an unfavourable increase of fat levels, which in the long run can give rise to arterial diseases, such as atherosclerosis.

On the other hand, when the men had to walk for 17,000 steps throughout the day, their bodies were able to break down the fat that was leftover in their bloodstreams – specifically the bad kind of fat that can lead to the development of cardiac disease (Finni et al., 2014). This emphasises the much greater role of having an active lifestyle with lots of movement throughout the entire day, as opposed to trying to counterbalance too much time spent sitting with short, intense bursts of exercise (Kim et al., 2016).

So what can we take away from all of this? We should look at exercise time and sedentary time as two entirely different entities. They are not as interconnected as we used to believe. Previously, public health programs and policies have primarily focused on the promotion of physical activity. This is probably misguided and doesn't reflect the most recent scientific findings. In light of risks that have been associated with a sedentary lifestyle, we need initiatives whose primary goal is to limit sitting time. However, such guidelines will only be effective if people are given the chance to put them into practice. Overarching environments, such as schools and offices, must be reorganised in a way that acknowledges our need to move. A wide spread restructuring in this regard, including the private and public sector, seems far away and will undoubtedly face considerable challenges. To be successful, we must change the old view that productive and meaningful work can only be achieved by an employee in front of a computer screen, seated at his or her desk.

SIT-STAND DESKS CANNOT
SOLVE OUR PROBLEMS

The introduction of height-adjustable desks in offices all over the world clearly reflects that there is a strong desire for health conscious work spaces. According to a 2017 survey by the Society for Human Resource Management, standing desks are the fastest growing benefits trend; 13% of employers provided or subsidised them in 2013 versus 44% in 2017.

So now the question becomes, can we cure this 'sitting disease' by elevating our desks? It would have been a shame if the solution had been this easy, and we had missed the corresponding health benefits over all these years. However, research has been done on the effects of the standing desk on our physiology, and the results have pointed towards some highly controversial issues.

One problem is that standing desks do not alleviate the detrimental effects on the metabolism, which are associated with inactivity. While not sitting, a standing person is still largely inactive. Many have altered their personal work environments in the effort to make a positive impact on their health, however, what they have gotten is an outright false sense of security that has not been backed by science.

The main issue with standing desks is connected to the very body position they force the user into. Standing for periods of time is unpleasant. Out of our own experience, we know that standing while waiting in a queue or behind a sales counter comes along with sensations of heaviness in the legs, back pain and generally leads to fatigue and even affects our mood.

Maintaining proper posture while standing in order to avoid the pain sensations described above proves to be challenging for many. There is a simple reason for this. Our human anatomy and physiology is not optimised to facilitate such a posture for any extended period of time. After years of sitting, the body's soft tissue and muscles have likely sustained considerable damage, resulting in relative weakness in the core and glute muscles, with consecutive lack of stabilisation and a forward tilted pelvis. Tight hip flexor muscles, which are often considerably shortened due to sitting, also contribute to a bad posture while standing. Same as in sitting, many people who stand tend to slouch and lean to one side, still relying rather loosely on soft tissue structures. The body easily comes off balance when standing, resulting in favouring one side or constant shifting forward and backward.

The posture typically seen in office workers using standing desks, is one where the arch in the lower back is exaggerated, resulting in compression of intervertebral disk spaces and often resulting in muscular pain. Lower back pain, therefore, is one of the most complaints that I have heard from patients using standing desks, which is somewhat ironic as many have sought to use standing desks to alleviate these same ailments.

What about the rest of the body? Our posture in the middle and upper portions of the back are not considerably changed when comparing standing to sitting. A forward bended head and neck posture in conjunction with rounded shoulders often contribute to pain in that area and spinal degeneration issues over time.

Scientific studies have looked into the question of standing desk

94

ergonomics. In a 2018 study, adult participants performed standing computer work to investigate possible changes in discomfort as well as cognitive function. After just two hours, most users complained of muscle fatigue, lower limb swelling and mental state deterioration, coupled with decreases in attention and reaction time (Baker et al., 2018).

The associated discomfort of height-adjustable desks often results in them not being used in the intended way. A large study performed in Germany looked at this question in more detail. Almost 700 participants were interviewed regarding their usage of a sit-to-stand desk. Out of the study population, 16% had access to such a desk, similar to the range of other countries. Surprisingly, only half of these individuals utilised the standing functionality of the desk, the remaining half had stopped standing and instead lowered it back to a height that allows usage with a conventional chair (Wallmann-Sperlich et al., 2017).

Having access to a standing desk also appears to fail in substantially decreasing overall sitting time, likely due to a compensation with more time spent inactive during leisure time. A systematic review that compared the results from 21 different trials, published in the Cochrane Registry in 2016, concluded that the availability of standing desks only leads to a reduction of overall sitting time of around 30 minutes to two hours (Shrestha et al., 2016).

This finding has greater implications when considering that a motivation for many users when starting to use a standing desk is the desire to lose body weight. To evaluate the potential a standing desk can contribute to such weight loss goals, it is interesting to look at an analysis of energy expenditure in sitting versus standing. This question has been addressed in numerous studies in the past. A large review published in Circulation in 2016 compared findings of 44 studies with more than 1,000 participants. What they found is that the mean difference in energy expenditure between sitting and standing was only 0.15kcal/min. This means, that if a user of a standing desk would theoretically use the desk exclusively for six hours per day nonstop, it would equate to around 50 additional burned calories (Saeidifard et al., 2016). An apple has around 100 calories, which means that an attempt to lose weight by using a standing desk is little more than wishful thinking

The question remains whether standing desks are actually good for our cardiac health or not. The predominant association is that standing workstations are measures to promote health in work environments. The existence of subsidised programs by health insurance companies also indicates their overall positive health benefits. However, looking into this further, we find that the latest research actually points in the opposite direction.

Standing for extended periods of time might actually cause more harm than good. A study from Canada compared standing and sitting at work across 7,000 workers; researchers reviewed the employees' healthcare records and looked for associations of occupational standing, sitting and cases of heart disease over the past 12 years. At the beginning of the study period, all of the people were free of heart disease. The study found that those who had to stand at their workplace had twice the risk of heart disease, compared to those who spent their time predominantly seated at work. Possible falsifying factors such as other health, sociodemographic, educational and work variables were excluded.

While not entirely understood, the underlying reasons are likely the result of a combination of too much blood pooling in the legs with an associated increase of pressure in the veins and an increase of oxidative stress in blood vessels. Over an extended period of time, this permanent stress on the vessel walls could explain the paradoxically increased risk for heart disease in those who stand more (Smith et al., 2017). And the heart doesn't appear to be the only organ that suffers from prolonged standing at work. Early studies have indicated that serious pregnancy related risks, such as preterm births and spontaneous abortions could also be a result (McCulloch et al., 2002, Waters et al, 2015).

EPILOGUE

WALKING TOWARDS THE FUTURE

The explosion of knowledge in medicine and the life sciences makes this some of the most exciting times we could ever imagine living in. As a species, we can expect to profit profoundly from the iterative exploration of new frontiers in medicine for years to come. An ever-widening holistic and scientific backed understanding of human health has swept away otherwise established beliefs with unprecedented speed and power.

Along with technologically facilitated democratisation, the accessibility of knowledge, and the possibility of understanding and interpreting personal health data, comes an ever faster progression towards improving one's own longevity and health span. Not only is this inevitable, it is already becoming a reality by many measures. Today's entrepreneurs have the ability to disrupt formerly unimaginable markets and continue to deliver smarter healthcare solutions to society's most pressing problems. And they'll do this by taking a lesson from the past, and then throwing tradition out the window.

The massive amount of accumulating evidence that relates inactivity and sedentariness to very real and concerning health risks can no longer be ignored. Socioeconomic pressure, resulting from exploding healthcare costs of chronic diseases linked to extended sitting, will also contribute to a faster implementation of countermeasures.

Thanks to immediate access to research data, rapid sharing through social media, and the resulting increase in public awareness, we will continue to see more profound changes fueled by growing pressure on policy makers. Inaction will simply no longer be an option, particularly once individuals link their own personal health with current political or corporate decisions. Our voting is often driven by our own experiences, and health issues related to sitting will continue to be felt by many.

Looking towards the next generation, Millennials already tend to favour work-life balance over career advancement or income, and personal health and mental wellbeing rank higher in life decision-making than ever before. Companies, cities, and nations as a whole will be driven to create better settings for their workforce and citizens, in which our fundamental health needs are best met.

So what should we expect? Generally, only tangible effort is able to transform knowledge and ideas into change. As such, if we want to see any meaningful difference, then it's up to us to take action. We must seek to overcome any existing barriers that are preventing us from living our healthiest and most enjoyable lives. The same is true for our urban architecture. It is us, the people, who will ultimately decide the direction that the future takes us.

Thankfully, there are many leaders at the corporate, municipality and government level who are changing the way we think about the world, and are dedicated to creating places in which the need for movement can unfold as our genetic code demands.

Limeade is a software company based in Bellevue, WA. Their product is an employee engagement platform that can be summarised with "bringing hearts and minds to work." This highly innovative company, headed by CEO Henry Albrecht, takes a pioneering role in exploring and researching what employees actually want from their workplace and how their engagement brings invaluable benefits for the companies' goals at the same time. And Limeade certainly practices what they preach. Every aspect of their headquarters has been meticulously designed to foster creativity and innovation; employees can use treadmill and bike desks, take naps, use mini trampolines or have flash fitness workouts all while keeping track of their steps with a free FitBit given to every employee. Limeade also heavily engages in proving the success of their methods through scientific studies and by measuring the impact of their software-enabled initiatives.

Copenhagen's Mayor, Frank Jensen, is another example of a leader who recognises the changing needs of our society, and his actions have been supported by impressive economic numbers. Leading the city since 2010, Jensen was named the world's second best politician by the FDI Association in 2013. He continuously finds ways to promote the attractiveness of Denmark's capital and has made the city the most bicycle-friendly and, by many statistics, the most eco-friendly in the world. Copenhagen's success lies in combining their green leadership with long-term, stable economic growth, making it highly attractive for businesses and investors. The relatively small city is one of the most productive in the world, with a gross value of over 83,000 USD per worker. At the same time, reports of life quality, life expectancy, happiness, social freedom and security rank the city amongst the top year after year.

What can we expect from continued technological advancement? The unparalleled success of wearables illustrates the appreciation and demand we have for assistance with everyday health related guidance and decision-making. Lasting habits are a result of availability, ease of use, and recognisable change. Wearables cater perfectly to these demands. The worldwide wearables market in 2017 reached 115.4 million units, up 10.3% from the 104.6 million units shipped in 2016. We can also expect to have affordable access to ever more advanced self-tracking technology in the near future, such as real time muscle blood perfusion and oxygen level measurement.

It can be easy to take this wealth of readily available and cost effective data for granted. Gaining so much information would have previously taken a dedicated research team. With this new collection of self-knowledge, we have the tools to re-shape our homes – and, in particular, our workplaces – to best align with our changing needs throughout the day. By receiving robust real time feedback right on our wrists, about how our current actions are affecting our health in a given moment, we simply don't have to wait for the results of expensive studies to be analysed before being published years later. Instead, we can conduct our very own studies, draw our own conclusions, and even contribute to studies with the data stored in our tracking devices.

How all of this will affect and shape the future workplace remains to be seen, though it will ultimately depend on what proves to have mutual benefits. One vivid new area in the field of office wellness is the way to stimulate all our senses in favour of optimising awareness, concentration and creativity through smart lighting and even auditory and olfactory measures. The overall concept of this is to bring vital natural elements back to our senses by applying neuroscientific findings in workplace settings.

Probably the two most important areas that we should expect to see reduced sedentary time in the years to come are transportation and – as discussed – office designs.

Next to our private homes, for which we are in charge, these two fields by far constitute the highest amount of sitting time at present. With the advent of self-driving vehicles, design thinkers will have the freedom to introduce entirely reimagined interior setups, which could enable us to reduce sitting time while commuting, with the potential of making significant daily impact.

When thinking about office workplaces, one of the most constant variables has been the need for any kind of desk. Prior to the advent of personal computers and typewriters, we required desks to handle paper and a surface to write on. While changing many aspects of how we work, smartphones and tablets have not yet reached their potential to truly provide the same degree of productivity for many types of work as a desktop computer. While the technology isn't there just yet, next generation headsets providing distraction free Augmented Reality / Virtual Reality could potentially make a desk unnecessary in the first place, giving us the ability to interact with complex data in a more productive and pleasurable way.

There is something bigger, which doesn't require the need for any kind of futuristic technology, and that is our ability to use our physical bodies to reach a mountain top in the sunrise or jog along a beach. I consider regular access to nature to be one of the most vital necessities for us as humans. While we set out to shape our workplaces and cities to meet our rediscovered needs, we should all strive for ways to spend quality time outside and plant this seed in the heads of our children early on. In the end, we are born movers because nature has shaped us in that way. Therefore, the journey ahead is at the same time a journey back to nature. I am excited with what we will make out of it.

REFERENCES

Aadahl, M., Kjaer, M., & Jørgensen, T. (2007). Influence of time spent on TV viewing and vigorous intensity physical activity on cardiovascular biomarkers. The Inter 99 study. Eur J Cardiovasc Prev Rehabil, Oct;14(5):660-5.

Abedi, P., Nikkhah, P., & Najar, S. (2015). Effect of pedometer-based walking on depression, anxiety and insomnia among postmenopausal women. Climacteric, 18(6):841-5.

Aldao, A., Dixon-Gordon, K.L., De Los Reyes, A. (2016). Individual differences in physiological flexibility predict spontaneous avoidance. Cogn Emot, Aug;30(5):985-98.

Alderman, B.L., Olson, R.L., Mattina, D.M. (2014). Cognitive function during low-intensity walking: a test of the treadmill workstation. J Phys Act Health, May;11(4):752-8.

Alesi, M., Bianco, A., Padulo, J., et al. (2014). Motor and cognitive development: the role of karate. Muscles Ligaments Tendons J., Apr; 4(2):114-20.

Alhowimel, A., AlOtaibi, M., Radford, K., & Coulson, N. (2018). Psychosocial factors associated with change in pain and disability outcomes in chronic low back pain patients treated by physiotherapist: A systematic review. SAGE Open Med, Feb 6;6:2050312118757387.

Alperovitch-Najenson, D., Santo, Y., Masharawi, Y., et al. (2010). Low back pain among professional bus drivers: ergonomic and occupational-psychosocial risk factors. Isr Med Assoc J, Jan;12(1):26-31.

Alzheimer's Disease International. Dementia Statistics. Accessed May 2018. Available: https://www.alz.co.uk/research/statistics.

American Diabetes Association (ADA). Statistics About Diabetes. Last Edited: March 22, 2018. Accessed March 2018. Available: http://www.diabetes.org/diabetes-basics/statistics/.

Anderssen, G.B.J. (1999). Epidemiologic features of chronic low back pain. Lancet, 354:581-5.

Arrieta, H., Rezola-Pardo, C., Echeverria, I., et al. (2018). Physical activity and fitness are associated with verbal memory, quality of life and depression among nursing home residents: preliminary data of a randomized controlled trial. BMC Geriatr, Mar 27;18(1):80.

Ashley, F., Kannel, W.B., Sorlie, P.D., & Masson, R. (1975). Pulmonary function: relation to aging, cigarette habit, and mortality. Ann Intern Med, Jun;82(6):739-45.

Azizbeigi, K., Stannard, S.R., Atashak, S., & Mosalman Haghighi, M. (2014). Antioxidant enzymes and oxidative stress adaptation to exercise training: Comparison of endurance, resistance, and concurrent training in untrained males. Journal of Exercise Science & Fitness, June;12(1):1-6.

Baker, Richelle, et al. "A detailed description of the short-term musculoskeletal and cognitive effects of prolonged standing for office computer work." Ergonomics 61.7 (2018): 877-890.

Balboa-Castillo, T., León-Muñoz, L.M., Graciani, A., et al. (2011). Longitudinal association of physical activity and sedentary behavior during leisure time with health-related quality of life in community-dwelling older adults. Health Qual Life Outcomes, Jun 27;9:47.

Baniqued, P.L., Gallen, C.L., Voss, M.W., et al. (2018). Brain Network Modularity Predicts Exercise-Related Executive Function Gains in Older Adults. Front Aging Neurosci, Jan 4;9:426.

Bär, K.J., Herbsleb, M., Schumann, A., et al. (2016). Hippocampal-Brainstem Connectivity Associated with Vagal Modulation after an Intense Exercise Intervention in Healthy Men. Front Neurosci, Apr 7;10:145.

Barton, W., Penney, N.C., Cronin, O., et al. (2018). The microbiome of professional athletes differs from that of more sedentary subjects in composition and particularly at the functional metabolic level. Gut, Apr;67(4):625-633.

Beckett, M.W., Ardern, C.I., & Rotondi, M.A. (2015). A meta-analysis of prospective studies on the role of physical activity and the prevention of Alzheimer's disease in older adults. BMC Geriatr, Feb 11;15:9.

Belcher, B.R., Berrigan, D., Papachristopoulou, A., et al. (2015). Effects of Interrupting Children's Sedentary Behaviors With Activity on Metabolic Function: A Randomized Trial. The Journal of Clinical Endocrinology and Metabolism, 100(10):3735–3743.

Bellon, K., Kolakowsky-Hayner, S., Wright, J., et al. (2015). A home-based walking study to ameliorate perceived stress and depressive symptoms in people with a traumatic brain injury. Brain Inj, 29(3):313-9.

Bernard, P., Ninot, G., Bernard, P.L., et al. (2015). Effects of a six-month walking intervention on depression in inactive post-menopausal women: a randomized controlled trial. Aging Ment Health, 19(6):485-92.

Bey, L, & Hamilton, M.T. (2003). Suppression of skeletal muscle lipoprotein lipase activity during physical inactivity: a molecular reason to maintain daily low-intensity activity. J Physiol, Sep 1; 551(Pt 2):673-82.

Biswas, Aviroop, et al. "Sedentary time and its association with risk for disease incidence, mortality, and hospitalization in adults: a systematic review and meta-analysis." Annals of internal medicine 162.2 (2015): 123-132.

Blackmore, D.G., Golmohammadi, M.G., Large, B., et al. (2009). Exercise increases neural stem cell number in a growth hormone-dependent manner, augmenting the regenerative response in aged mice. Stem Cells, Aug;27(8):2044-52.

Bloom, D.E., Cafiero, E.T., Jané-Llopis, E., et al. (2011). The global economic burden of noncommunicable diseases (Working Paper Series). Geneva: Harvard School of Public Health and World Economic Forum.

Blumenthal, J.A., Williams, R.S., Needels, T.L., & Wallace, A.G. (1982). Psychological changes accompany aerobic exercise in healthy middle-aged adults. Psychosom Med, Dec;44(6):529-36.

Blumenthal, J. A., Sherwood, A., Babyak, M. A., et al. (2012). Exercise and Pharmacological Treatment of Depressive Symptoms in Patients with Coronary Heart Disease: Results from the UPBEAT Study. Journal of the American College of Cardiology, 60(12):1053–1063.

Bonaz, B., Sinniger, V., & Pellissier, S. (2016). Vagal tone: effects on sensitivity, motility, and inflammation. Neurogastroenterol Motil, Apr;28(4):455-62.

Bondy, C.A., & Cheng, C.M. (2004). Review Signaling by insulin-like growth factor 1 in brain. Eur J Pharmacol, Apr 19; 490(1-3):25-31.

Breit, S., Kupferberg, A., Rogler, G., & Hasler, G. (2018). Vagus Nerve as Modulator of the Brain-Gut Axis in Psychiatric and Inflammatory Disorders. Front Psychiatry, Mar 13;9:44.

Brinkmann, C., Schäfer, L., Masoud, M., et al. (2017). Effects of Cycling and Exergaming on Neurotrophic Factors in Elderly Type 2 Diabetic Men - A Preliminary Investigation. Exp Clin Endocrinol Diabetes, Jul;125(7):436-440.

Brinton, L.A., Cook, M.B., McCormack, V., et al. (2014). Anthropometric and hormonal risk factors for male breast cancer: male breast cancer pooling project results. Journal of the National Cancer Institute, 106(3):djt465.

Campbell, P.T., Newton, C.C., Freedman, N.D., et al. (2016). Body mass index, waist circumference, diabetes, and risk of liver cancer for U.S. adults. Cancer Research, 76(20):6076-6083.

Canadian Diabetes Association. (2009). Economic Tsunami: The Cost of Diabetes in America. Accessed March 2018. Available: https://www.diabetes.ca/CDA/media/documents/publications-and-newsletters/advocacy-reports/economic-tsunami-cost-of-diabetes-in-canada-english.pdf.

Carro, E., Trejo, J.L., Busiguina, S., & Torres-Aleman, I. (2001). Circulating insulin-like growth factor I mediates the protective effects of physical exercise against brain insults of different etiology and anatomy. J Neurosci, Aug 1;21(15):5678-84.

Castelli, D.M., Hillman, C.H., Buck, S.M., & Erwin, H.E. (2007). Physical fitness and academic achievement in third- and fifth-grade students. J Sport Exerc Psychol, Apr; 29(2):239-52.

Cawley, J., & Meyerhoefer, C. (2012). The Medical Care Costs of Obesity: An Instrumental Variables Approach. Journal of Health Economics, 31(1): 219-230.

Cawley, J., Rizzo, J.A., & Haas, K. (2007). Occupation-specific Absenteeism Costs Associated with Obesity and Morbid Obesity. Journal of Occupational and Environmental Medicine, 49(12):1317?24.

Celik, S., Celik, K., Dirimese, E., et al. (2018). Determination of pain in musculoskeletal system reported by office workers and the pain risk factors. Int J Occup Med Environ Health, Jan 1;31(1):91-111.

Chandwani, H.S. (2013). The economic burden of chronic back pain in the United States: a societal perspective. Accessed March 2018. Available: https://repositories.lib.utexas.edu/handle/2152/23087.

Chastin, S.F., Culhane, B., Dall, P.M. (2014). Comparison of self-reported measure of sitting time (IPAQ) with objective measurement (activPAL). Physiol Meas, 35:2319–2328.

Chen, Y., Liu, L., Wang, X., et al. (2013). Body mass index and risk of gastric cancer: a meta-analysis of a population with more than ten million from 24 prospective studies. Cancer Epidemiology, Biomarkers & Prevention, 22(8):1395-1408.

Chen, Y., Wang, X., Wang, J., et al. (2012). Excess body weight and the risk of primary liver cancer: an updated meta-analysis of prospective studies. European Journal of Cancer, 48(14):2137-2145.

Chirchir, H., Ruff, C.B., Junno, J.A., & Potts, R. (2017). Low trabecular bone density in recent sedentary modern humans. Am J Phys Anthropol, Mar;162(3):550-560.

Cho, J.W., Jung, S.Y., Lee, S.W., et al. (2017). Treadmill exercise ameliorates social isolation-induced depression through neuronal generation in rat pups. J Exerc Rehabil, Dec 27;13(6):627-633.

Chomitz, V.R., Slining, M.M., McGowan, R.J., et al. (2009). Is there a relationship between physical fitness and academic achievement? Positive results from public school children in the northeastern United States. J Sch

Health, Jan; 79(1):30-7.

Clarke, S.F., Murphy, E.F., O'Sullivan, O., et al. (2014). Exercise and associated dietary extremes impact on gut microbial diversity. Gut, Dec; 63(12):1913-20.

Clemes, S.A., Patel, R., Mahon, C., & Griffiths, P.L. (2014). Sitting time and step counts in office workers. Occup Med (Lond), Apr;64(3):188-92.

Colcombe, S.J., Kramer, A.F., Erickson, K.I., et al. (2004). Cardiovascular fitness, cortical plasticity, and aging. Proc Natl Acad Sci U S A., Mar 2; 101(9):3316-21.

Colcombe, S.J., Erickson, K.I., Scalf, P.E., et al. (2006). Aerobic exercise training increases brain volume in aging humans. J Gerontol A Biol Sci Med Sci, Nov; 61(11):1166-70.

Collaborative Group on Epidemiological Studies of Ovarian Cancer. (2012). Ovarian cancer and body size: individual participant meta-analysis including 25,157 women with ovarian cancer from 47 epidemiological studies. PLoS Medicine, 9(4):e1001200.

CPWR - The Center for Construction Research and Training. (2002). CPWR Technical Report: Analysis of Work-Related Safety & Health Hazards of Unrepresented Workers in the Iron Working Industry. Feb 2010. Accessed March 2018. Available: http://www.elcosh.org/document/2055/d001031/CPWR+Technical+Report:+Analysis+of+Work-Related+Safety+&+Health+Hazards+of+Unrepresented+Workers+in+the+Iron+Working+Industry.html.

Cronin, O., Barton, W., Skuse, P., et al. (2018). A Prospective Metagenomic and Metabolomic Analysis of the Impact of Exercise and/or Whey Protein Supplementation on the Gut Microbiome of Sedentary Adults. mSystems, Apr 24;3(3).

Crosbie, W.J., & Myles, S. (1985). An investigation into effect of postural modification on some aspect of normal pulmonary function. Physiotherapy, 71:311-314.

Crush, E.A., Frith, E., & Loprinzi, P.D. (2018). Experimental effects of acute exercise duration and exercise recovery on mood state. J Affect Disord, Mar 15;229:282-287.

Cui, M.Y., Lin, Y., Sheng, J.Y., et al. (2018). Exercise Intervention Associated with Cognitive Improvement in Alzheimer's Disease. Neural Plast, Mar 11;2018:9234105.

Dagenais, S., Caro, J., Haldeman, S. (2008). A systematic review of low back pain cost of illness studies in the United States and internationally. Spine J., Jan-Feb;8(1):8-20.

Dalla, C., Papachristos, E.B., Whetstone, A.S., & Shors, T.J. (2009). Female rats learn trace memories better than male rats and consequently retain a greater proportion of new neurons in their hippocampi. Proc Natl Acad Sci U S A., Feb 24; 106(8):2927-32.

DeFina, L.F., Willis, B.L., Radford, N.B., et al. (2013). The Association Between Midlife Cardiorespiratory Fitness Levels and Later-Life Dementia: A Cohort Study. Annals of Internal Medicine, 158(3):162–168.

Dempsey, P.C., Dunstan, D.W., Larsen, R.N., et al. (2018). Prolonged uninterrupted sitting increases fatigue in type 2 diabetes. Diabetes Res Clin Pract, Jan;135:128-133.

Department of Health. (2007). Improving diabetes services: the NSF four years on. Accessed April 2018. Available: www.dvh.nhs.uk/downloads/documents/B81F82BI76_the_way_ahead_th e_local_challenge.pdf.

Després, J.P. (2007). Cardiovascular disease under the influence of excess visceral fat. Crit Pathw Cardiol, Jun;6(2):51-9.

Deyo, R.A., Von Korff, M., & Duhrkoop, D. (2015). Opioids for low back pain. BMJ, Jan 5;350:g6380.

Diabetes UK. (2010). Diabetes in the UK 2010: Key statistics on diabetes - published March 2010. Accessed April 2018. Available: https://www.diabetes.org.uk/resources-s3/2017-11/diabetes_in_the_uk_2010.pdf.

Diaz, K.M., Howard, V.J., Hutto, B., (2017). Patterns of Sedentary Behavior and Mortality in U.S. Middle-Aged and Older Adults. Ann Intern Med, Oct 3;167(7):465-475.

Ding, Y.H., Li, J., Zhou, Y., et al. (2006). Cerebral angiogenesis and expression of angiogenic factors in aging rats after exercise. Curr Neurovasc Res, Feb; 3(1):15-23.

Ding, K., Tarumi, T., Zhu, D.C., et al. (2018). Cardiorespiratory Fitness and White Matter Neuronal Fiber Integrity in Mild Cognitive Impairment. J Alzheimers Dis, 61(2):729-739.

Dobbs, R., Sawers, C., Thompson, F., et al. (2014). Overcoming Obesity: An Initial Economic Analysis. McKinsey Global Institute; Jakarta, Indonesia.

Doose, M., Ziegenbein, M., Hoos, O., et al. (2015). Self-selected intensity exercise in the treatment of major depression: A pragmatic RCT. Int J Psychiatry Clin Pract, 19(4):266-75.

Dougan, M.M., Hankinson, S.E., Vivo, I.D., et al. (2015). Prospective study of body size throughout the life-course and the incidence of endometrial cancer among premenopausal and postmenopausal women. International Journal of Cancer, 137(3):625-37.

Drenowatz, C., DeMello, M.M., Shook, R.P., et al. (2016). The association between sedentary behaviors during weekdays and weekend with change in body composition in young adults. AIMS Public Health, Jun 3;3(2):375-388.

Dunbar, C.C., & Kalinski, M.I. (1994). Cardiac intracellular regulation: exercise effects on the cAMP system and A-kinase. Med Sci Sports Exerc, Dec;26(12):1459-65.

Dunlop, D.D., Song, J., Arntson, E.K., et al. (2015). Sedentary time in U.S. older adults associated with disability in activities of daily living independent of physical activity. Journal of Physical Activity & Health, 12(1), 93–101.

Dunn, J.P., Cowan, R.L., Volkow, N.D., et al. (2010). Decreased dopamine type 2 receptor availability after bariatric surgery: preliminary findings. Brain Res, Sep 2; 1350:123-30.

Duvivier, B.M., Schaper, N.C., Hesselink, M.K., et al. (2017). Breaking sitting with light activities vs structured exercise: a randomised crossover study demonstrating benefits for glycaemic control and insulin sensitivity in type 2 diabetes. Diabetologia, Mar;60(3):490-498.

Egan, M.F., Kojima, M., Callicott, J.H., et al. (2003). The BDNF val66met polymorphism affects activity-dependent secretion of BDNF and human memory and hippocampal function. Cell, Jan 24; 112(2):257-69.

Ehmann, P.J., Brush, C.J., Olson, R.L., et al. (2017). Active Workstations Do Not Impair Executive Function in Young and Middle-Age Adults. Med Sci Sports Exerc, May;49(5):965-974.

Ekelund, Ulf, et al. "Does physical activity attenuate, or even eliminate, the detrimental association of sitting time with mortality? A harmonised meta-analysis of data from more than 1 million men and women." The Lancet 388.10051 (2016): 1302-1310.

Ensari, I., Sandroff, B.M., & Motl, R.W. (2017). Intensity of treadmill walking exercise on acute mood symptoms in persons with multiple sclerosis. Anxiety Stress Coping, Jan;30(1):15-25.

Fabbrini, E., Sullivan, S., & Klein, S. (2010). Obesity and nonalcoholic fatty liver disease: Biochemical, metabolic and clinical implications. Hepatology, 51:679–689.

Ferland, A., Château-Degat, M.L., Hernandez, T.L., & Eckel, R.H. (2012). Tissue-specific responses of lipoprotein lipase to dietary macronutrient composition as a predictor of weight gain over 4 years. Obesity (Silver Spring), May;20(5):1006-11.

Ferris, L.T., Williams, J.S., & Shen, C.L. (2007). The effect of acute exercise on serum brain-derived neurotrophic factor levels and cognitive function. Med Sci Sports Exerc, Apr; 39(4):728-34.

Filliau, C., Younes, M., Blanchard, A.L., et al. (2015). Effect of "Touch Rugby" Training on the Cardiovascular Autonomic Control In Sedentary Subjects. Int J Sports Med, Jun;36(7):567-72.

Finni, T., et al. "Exercise for fitness does not decrease the muscular inactivity time during normal daily life." Scandinavian journal of medicine & science in sports 24.1 (2014): 211-219.

Fisher, B.E., Li, Q., Nacca, A., Salem, G.J., et al. (2013). Treadmill exercise elevates striatal dopamine D2 receptor binding potential in patients with early Parkinson's disease. Neuroreport, Jul 10;24(10):509-14.

Ford, E.S., & Caspersen, C.J. (2012). Sedentary behaviour and cardiovascular disease: a review of prospective studies. Int J Epidemiol, Oct;41(5):1338-53.

Frischenschlager, E., & Gosch, J. (2012).. Active Learning—Leichter lernen durch Bewegung. [Active Learning—Easier learning through physical activity] Erzieh. Unterr, 162:131–137.

Froy, O. (2010). Metabolism and Circadian Rhythms—Implications for Obesity. Endocrine Reviews, Feb 1, 31(1):1–24.

Fujii, T., Oka, H., Katsuhira, J., et al. (2018). Association between somatic symptom burden and health-related quality of life in people with chronic low back pain. PLoS One, Feb 20;13(2):e0193208.

Fuss, J., Steinle, J., Bindila, L., et al. (2015). A runner's high depends on cannabinoid receptors in mice. Proc Natl Acad Sci U S A., Oct 20; 112(42):13105-8.

Gallagher, D., Terenzi, T., de Meersman, R. (1992). Heart rate variability in smokers, sedentary and aerobically fit individuals. Clin Auton Res, Dec;2(6):383-7.

Gallagher, E.J., LeRoith, D. (2015). Obesity and diabetes: The increased risk of cancer and cancer-related mortality. Physiological Reviews, 95(3):727-748.

Genkinger, J.M., Spiegelman, D., Anderson, K.E., et al. (2011). A pooled analysis of 14 cohort studies of anthropometric factors and pancreatic cancer risk. International Journal of Cancer, 129(7):1708-1717.

Gilson, N.D., Hall, C., Renton, A., et al. (2017). Do Sitting, Standing, or Treadmill Desks Impact Psychobiological Indicators of Work Productivity? J Phys Act Health, Oct 1;14(10):793-796.

Gokal, K., Wallis, D., Ahmed, S., et al. (2016). Effects of a self-managed home-based walking intervention on psychosocial health outcomes for breast cancer patients receiving chemotherapy: a randomised controlled trial. Support Care Cancer, Mar;24(3):1139-66.

Gordon-Larsen, P., Hou, N., Sidney, S., et al. (2009). Fifteen-year longitudinal trends in walking patterns and their impact on weight change. Am J Clin Nutr, Jan;89(1):19-26.

Gourgouvelis, J., Yielder, P., Clarke, S.T., et al. (2018). Exercise Leads to Better Clinical Outcomes in Those Receiving Medication Plus Cognitive

Behavioral Therapy for Major Depressive Disorder. Front Psychiatry, Mar 6;9:37.

Gregor, M.F., & Hotamisligil, G.S. (2011). Inflammatory mechanisms in obesity. Annual Review of Immunology, 29:415-445.

Guiraud, T., Labrunee, M., Gaucher-Cazalis, K., et al. (2013). High-intensity interval exercise improves vagal tone and decreases arrhythmias in chronic heart failure. Med Sci Sports Exerc, Oct;45(10):1861-7.

Gunter, M.J., Hoover, D.R., Yu, H., et al. (2008). A prospective evaluation of insulin and insulin-like growth factor-I as risk factors for endometrial cancer. Cancer Epidemiol Biomarkers Prev, Apr;17(4):921-9.

Guo, X., Pantoni, L., Simoni, M., et al. (2006). Midlife respiratory function related to white matter lesions and lacunar infarcts in late life: the Prospective Population Study of Women in Gothenburg, Sweden. Stroke, Jul;37(7):1658-62.

Gustafsson, E., Johnson, P.W., & Hagberg, M., (2010), Thumb postures and physical loads during mobile phone use - a comparison of young adults with and without musculoskeletal symptoms. J Electromyogr Kinesiol, 20(1):127-35.

Hallam, K.T., Bilsborough, S., & de Courten, M. (2018). "Happy feet": evaluating the benefits of a 100-day 10,000 step challenge on mental health and wellbeing. BMC Psychiatry, Jan 24;18(1):19.

Hamer, M., & Chida, Y. (2008). Walking and primary prevention: a meta-analysis of prospective cohort studies. Br J Sports Med, Apr;42(4):238-43.
Hamilton, A.M.P., Ulbig, M.W., & Polkinghorne, P. (1996). Management of diabetic retinopathy, London: BMJ Publishing.

Hamilton, M.T., Areiqat, E., Hamilton, D.G., & Bey, L. (2001). Plasma triglyceride metabolism in humans and rats during aging and physical inactivity. Int J Sport Nutr Exerc Metab, Dec;11 Suppl:S97-104.

Hamilton, M.T., Hamilton, D.G., Zderic, T.W. (2007). Role of low energy expenditure and sitting in obesity, metabolic syndrome, type 2 diabetes, and cardiovascular disease. Diabetes, Nov;56(11):2655-67.

Hancox, R.J., Poulton, R., Greene, J.M., et al. (2007). Systemic inflammation and lung function in young adults. Thorax, 62(12):1064–1068.

Hariri, A.R., Goldberg, T.E., Mattay, V.S., et al. (2003). Brain-derived neurotrophic factor val66met polymorphism affects human memory-related hippocampal activity and predicts memory performance. J Neurosci, Jul 30;23(17):6690-4.

Hartescu, I., Morgan, K., Stevinson, C.D. (2015). Increased physical activity improves sleep and mood outcomes in inactive people with insomnia: a randomized controlled trial. J Sleep Res, Oct;24(5):526-34.

Hatala, K.G., Demes, B., & Richmond, B.G. (2016). Laetoli footprints reveal bipedal gait biomechanics different from those of modern humans and chimpanzees. Proc Biol Sci, Aug 17;283(1836).

Hayashi, Tomoshige., et al. "High normal blood pressure, hypertension, and the risk of type 2 diabetes in Japanese men. The Osaka Health Survey." Diabetes Care 22.10 (1999): 1683-1687.

Hellsing, E. (1989). Changes in the pharyngeal airway in relation to extension of the head. Eur. J. Orthodol., 11:359-365.

Hillman, C.H., Pontifex, M.B., Castelli, D.M., et al. (2014). Effects of the FITKids Randomized Controlled Trial on Executive Control and Brain Function. Pediatrics, 134(4), e1063–e1071.

Holsinger, R.M., Schnarr, J., Henry, P., et al. (2000). Quantitation of BDNF mRNA in human parietal cortex by competitive reverse transcription-polymerase chain reaction: decreased levels in Alzheimer's disease. Brain Res Mol Brain Res, Mar 29; 76(2):347-54.

Hörder, H., Johansson, L., Guo, X., et al. (2018). Midlife cardiovascular fitness and dementia: A 44-year longitudinal population study in women. Neurology, Apr 10;90(15):e1298-e1305.

Howden, E.J., La Gerche, A., Arthur, J.F., et al. (2018). Standing up to the cardiometabolic consequences of hematological cancers. Blood Rev, Feb 21, pii: S0268-960X(17)30088-7.

Hoyo, C., Cook, M.B., Kamangar, F., et al. (2012). Body mass index in relation to oesophageal and oesophagogastric junction adenocarcinomas: a pooled analysis from the International BEACON Consortium. International Journal of Epidemiology, 41(6):1706-1718.

Hu, F.B., Stampfer, M.J., Colditz, G.A., et al. (2000). Physical activity and risk of stroke in women. JAMA, Jun 14;283(22):2961-7.

Hurwitz, E.L., Randhawa, K., Yu, H., Côté, P., & Haldeman, S. (2018). The Global Spine Care Initiative: a summary of the global burden of low back and neck pain studies. Eur Spine J, Feb 26. [Epub ahead of print].

Imbeault, P., Doucet, E., Mauriège, P., et al. (2001). Difference in leptin response to a high-fat meal between lean and obese men. Clin Sci (Lond), Oct;101(4):359-65.

International Diabetes Federation (IDF). (2013). IDF Diabetes Atlas, 6th ed. Brussels, online version of IDF Diabetes Atlas. Accessed April 2018. Available: www.idf.org/diabetesatlas.

Joubert, J., Norman, R., Bradshaw, D., et al. (2007). Estimating the burden of disease attributable to excess body weight in South Africa in 2000. South African Med J, 97(8):683–90.

Kaaks, R., Lukanova, A., Kurzer, M.S. (2002). Obesity, endogenous hormones, and endometrial cancer risk: a synthetic review. Cancer Epidemiol Biomark Prev, 11:1531-43.

Kamijo, K., O'Leary, K.C., Pontifex, M.B., et al. (2010). The relation of aerobic fitness to neuroelectric indices of cognitive and motor task preparation. Psychophysiology, Sep;47(5):814-21.

Kang, H.K., Park, H.Y., Jeong, B.H., et al. (2015). Relationship Between Forced Vital Capacity and Framingham Cardiovascular Risk Score Beyond the Presence of Metabolic Syndrome: The Fourth Korea National Health and Nutrition Examination Survey. Medicine (Baltimore), Nov;94(47):e2089.

Kapreli, E., Vourazanis, E., Strimpakos, N. (2008). Neck pain causes respiratory dysfunction. Med Hypotheses, 70(5):1009-13.

Kerling, A., Kück, M., Tegtbur, U., et al. (2017). Exercise increases serum brain-derived neurotrophic factor in patients with major depressive disorder. J Affect Disord, Jun;215:152-155.

Kiecolt-Glaser, J.K., Derry, H.M., & Fagundes, C.P.. (2015). Inflammation: depression fans the flames and feasts on the heat. Am J Psychiatry, Nov 1;172(11):1075-91.

Kim, H., Min, T.J., Kang, S.H., et al. (2017). Association Between Walking and Low Back Pain in the Korean Population: A Cross-Sectional Study. Ann Rehabil Med, Oct;41(5):786-792.

Kitahara, C.M., Platz, E.A., Freeman, L.E., et al. (2011). Obesity and thyroid cancer risk among US men and women: A pooled analysis of five prospective studies. Cancer Epidemiol. Biomarkers Prev, 20:464–472.

Klyne, D.M., Barbe, M.F., van den Hoorn, W., & Hodges, P.W. (2018). ISSLS PRIZE IN CLINICAL SCIENCE 2018: longitudinal analysis of inflammatory, psychological, and sleep-related factors following an acute low back pain episode-the good, the bad, and the ugly. Eur Spine J, Feb 19. [Epub ahead of print].

Knott, C.S., Panter, J., Foley, L., & Ogilvie, D. (2018). Changes in the mode of travel to work and the severity of depressive symptoms: a longitudinal analysis of UK Biobank. Prev Med, Mar 28;112:61-69.

Knowler, W.C., Barrett-Connor, E., Fowler, S.E., et al. (2002). Reduction in the incidence of type 2 diabetes with lifestyle intervention or metformin. N Engl J Med, Feb 7; 346(6):393-403.

Kochi, C., Liu, H., Zaidi, S., et al. (2017). Prior treadmill exercise promotes resilience to vicarious trauma in rats. Prog Neuropsychopharmacol Biol Psychiatry, Jul 3;77:216-221.

Kolaczynski, J.W., Nyce, M.R., Considine, R.V., et al. (1996). Acute and chronic effects of insulin on leptin production in humans: Studies in vivo and in vitro. Diabetes, May;45(5):699-701.

Korzeniowska-Kubacka, I., Bilinska, M., Piotrowska, D., et al. (2017). The impact of exercise-only-based rehabilitation on depression and anxiety in patients after myocardial infarction. Eur J Cardiovasc Nurs, Jun;16(5):390-396.

Kowianski, P., Lietzau, G., Czuba, E., et al. (2018). BDNF: A Key Factor with Multipotent Impact on Brain Signaling and Synaptic Plasticity. Cellular and Molecular Neurobiology, 38(3):579–593.

Kravitz, A.V., O'Neal, T.J., & Friend, D.M. (2016). Do Dopaminergic Impairments Underlie Physical Inactivity in People with Obesity? Frontiers in Human Neuroscience, 10:514.

Kulmala, J., Solomon, A., Kåreholt, I., et al. (2014). Association between mid- to late life physical fitness and dementia: evidence from the CAIDE study. J Intern Med, Sep;276(3):296-307.

Kwan, M.L., Kroenke, C.H., Sweeney, C., et al. (2015). Association of high obesity with PAM50 breast cancer intrinsic subtypes and gene expression. BMC Cancer, Apr 14;15:278.

Kim, Il-Young, et al. "Prolonged sitting negatively affects the postprandial plasma triglyceride-lowering effect of acute exercise." American Journal of Physiology-Endocrinology and Metabolism 311.5 (2016): E891-E898.

Labelle, H., Roussouly, P., Berthonnaud, E., et al. (2005). The importance of spino-pelvic balance in L5-s1 developmental spondylolisthesis: a review of pertinent radiologic measurements. Spine (Phila Pa 1976), Mar 15;30(6 Suppl):S27-34.

LaCroix, A.Z., Leveille, S.G., Hecht, J.A., et al. (1996). Does walking decrease the risk of cardiovascular disease hospitalizations and death in older adults? J Am Geriatr Soc, 44:113-120.

Landers, M., Barker, G., Wallentine, S., et al. (2003). A comparison of tidal volume, breathing frequency, and minute ventilation between two sitting postures in healthy adults. Physiother. Theory Pract, 19:109-119.

Landolt, K., Maruff, P., Horan, B., et al. (2017). Chronic work stress and decreased vagal tone impairs decision making and reaction time in jockeys. Psychoneuroendocrinology, Oct;84:151-158.

Laricchiuta, D., Andolina, D., Angelucci, F., et al. (2018). Cerebellar BDNF Promotes Exploration and Seeking for Novelty. Int J Neuropsychopharmacol, May 1;21(5):485-498.

Larson, M.J., LeCheminant, J.D., Carbine, K., et al. (2015). Slow walking on a treadmill desk does not negatively affect executive abilities: an examination of cognitive control, conflict adaptation, response inhibition, and post-error slowing. Front Psychol, May 27;6:723.

Levine, J.A., & Miller, J.M. (2007). The energy expenditure of using a "walk-and-work" desk for office workers with obesity. British Journal of Sports Medicine, 41(9), 558–561.

Liao, D., Higgins, M., Bryan, N.R., et al. (1999). Lower pulmonary function and cerebral subclinical abnormalities detected by MRI: the Atherosclerosis Risk in Communities study. Chest, Jul;116(1):150-6.

Li, L., Gan, Y., Li, W., et al. (2016). Overweight, obesity and the risk of gallbladder and extrahepatic bile duct cancers: A meta-analysis of observational studies. Obesity (Silver Spring), 24(8):1786-1802.

Lichtman, M.A. (2010). Obesity and the risk for a hematological malignancy: Leukemia, lymphoma, or myeloma. Oncologist, 15:1083–1101.

Lin, F., Parthasarathy, S., i, S.J., et al. (2006). Effect of different sitting postures on lung capacity, expiratory flow, and lumbar lordosis. Arch Phys Med Rehabil, Apr;87(4):504-9.

Lin, I.M., & Peper, E., (2009), Psychophysiological patterns during cell phone text messaging: a preliminary study. Appl Psychophysiol Biofeedback, 34(1):53-7.

López-Cruz, L., San Miguel, N., Carratalá-Ros, C., et al. (2018). Dopamine depletion shifts behavior from activity based reinforcers to more sedentary ones and adenosine receptor antagonism reverses that shift: Relation to ventral striatum DARPP32 phosphorylation patterns. Neuropharmacology. 2018 Feb 2. pii: S0028-3908(18)30034-0. [Epub ahead of print].

Lorbergs, A.L., O'Connor, G.T., Zhou, Y., et al. (2017). Severity of Kyphosis and Decline in Lung Function: The Framingham Study. J Gerontol A Biol Sci Med Sci, May 1;72(5):689-694.

Ma, Q. (2008). Beneficial effects of moderate voluntary physical exercise and its biological mechanisms on brain health. Neurosci Bull, Aug;24(4):265-70.

Ma, Y., Yang, Y., Wang, F., et al. (2013). Obesity and risk of colorectal cancer: a systematic review of prospective studies. PLoS One, 8(1):e53916.

Ma, X., Yue, Z.-Q., Gong, Z.-Q., et al. (2017). The Effect of Diaphragmatic Breathing on Attention, Negative Affect and Stress in Healthy Adults. Frontiers in Psychology, 8:874.

McAllister, A.K., Katz, L.C., Lo, D.C. (1996). Neurotrophin regulation of cortical dendritic growth requires activity. Neuron, Dec;17(6):1057-64.

McCulloch, John. "Health risks associated with prolonged standing." Work 19.2 (2002): 201-205.

McDonald, M.L., MacMullen, C., Liu, D.J., et al. (2012). Genetic association of cyclic AMP signaling genes with bipolar disorder. Transl Psychiatry, Oct 2;2:e169.

MacEwen, B.T., MacDonald, D.J., Burr, J.F. (2015). Review A systematic review of standing and treadmill desks in the workplace. Prev Med, Jan; 70:50-8.

Mackay, C.P., Kuys, S.S., Brauer, S.G.. (2017). The Effect of Aerobic Exercise on Brain-Derived Neurotrophic Factor in People with Neurological Disorders: A Systematic Review and Meta-Analysis. Neural Plast, 2017:4716197.

McTiernan, A. (2008). Mechanisms linking physical activity with cancer. Nat Rev Cancer, Mar;8(3):205-11.

Maniadakis, N., & Gray, A. (2000). The economic burden of back pain in the UK. Pain, Feb, 84(1):95-103.

Manohar, C., Levine, J.A., Nandy, D.K., et al. (2012). The effect of walking on postprandial glycemic excursion in patients with type 1 diabetes and healthy people. Diabetes Care, Dec;35(12):2493-9.

Manson, J.E., Greenland, P., LaCroix, A.Z., et al. (2002). Walking compared with vigorous exercise for the prevention of cardiovascular events in women. N Engl J Med, 347:716–725.

Marchesini, G., Moscatiello, S., Di Domizio, S., & Forlani, G. (2008). Obesity-associated liver disease. J. Clin. Endocrinol. Metab, 93:S74–S80.

Marcourakis, T., Gorenstein, C., Brandão de Almeida Prado, E., et al. (2002). Panic disorder patients have reduced cyclic AMP in platelets. J Psychiatr Res, Mar-Apr;36(2):105-10.

Matthews, C.E., George, S.M., Moore, S.C., et al. (2012). Amount of time spent in sedentary behaviors and cause-specific mortality in US adults. Am J Clin Nutr, Feb;95(2):437-45.

Molteni, R., Ying, Z., Gómez-Pinilla, F. (2002). Differential effects of acute and chronic exercise on plasticity-related genes in the rat hippocampus revealed by microarray. Eur J Neurosci, Sep; 16(6):1107-16.

Morgan, J.A., Olagunju, A.T., Corrigan, F., & Baune, B.T. (2018). Does ceasing exercise induce depressive symptoms? A systematic review of experimental trials including immunological and neurogenic markers. J Affect Disord, Jul;234:180-192.

Morrish, N.J., Wang, S.L., Stevens, L.K., et al. (2001). Mortality and causes of death in the WHO: multinational study of vascular disease in diabetes. Diabetologia 44, suppl 2; s14–s21.

Mosconi, L., Pupi, A., De Leon, M.J. (2008). Review Brain glucose hypometabolism and oxidative stress in preclinical Alzheimer's disease. Ann N Y Acad Sci, Dec;1147:180-95.

Movius, H.L., & Allen, J.J. (2005). Cardiac Vagal Tone, defensiveness, and motivational style. Biol Psychol, Feb;68(2):147-62.

Munsell, M.F., Sprague, B.L., Berry, D.A., et al. (2014). Body mass index and breast cancer risk according to postmenopausal estrogen-progestin use and hormone receptor status. Epidemiologic Reviews, 36:114-136.

Ng, M., Fleming, T., Robinson, M., et al. (2013). Global, regional, and national prevalence of overweight and obesity in children and adults during 1980–2013: a systematic analysis for the Global Burden of Disease Study. Lancet, Aug 30;384(9945):766-81.

Niedermaier, T., Behrens, G., Schmid, D., et al. (2015). Body mass index, physical activity, and risk of adult meningioma and glioma: A meta-analysis. Neurology, 85(15):1342-1350.

Nyberg, J., Åberg, M.A., Schiöler, L., et al. (2014). Cardiovascular and cognitive fitness at age 18 and risk of early-onset dementia. Brain, May;137(Pt 5):1514-23.

Ojo, S.O., Bailey, D.P., Chater, A.M., & Hewson, D.J. (2018). The Impact of Active Workstations on Workplace Productivity and Performance: A Systematic Review. Int J Environ Res Public Health, Feb 27;15(3). pii: E417.

Olshansky, S.J., Passaro, D.J., Hershow, R.C., et al. (2005). A potential decline in life expectancy in the United States in the 21st century. N Engl J Med, Mar 17;352(11):1138-45.

Oppezzo, M., & Schwartz, D.L. (2014). Give your ideas some legs: the positive effect of walking on creative thinking. J Exp Psychol Learn Mem Cogn, Jul; 40(4):1142-52.

Orsini, N., Bellocco, R., Bottai, M., et al. (2009). A prospective study of lifetime physical activity and prostate cancer incidence and mortality. Br J Cancer, Dec 1;101(11):1932-8.

Ostermann, S., Herbsleb, M., Schulz, S., et al. (2013). Exercise reveals the interrelation of physical fitness, inflammatory response, psychopathology, and autonomic function in patients with schizophrenia. Schizophr Bull, Sep;39(5):1139-49.

O'Sullivan, O., Cronin, O., Clarke, S.F., et al. (2015). Exercise and the microbiota. Gut Microbes, 6(2):131-6.

Paret, L., Bailey, H.N., Roche, J., et al. (2015). Preschool ambivalent attachment associated with a lack of vagal withdrawal in response to stress. Attach Hum Dev, 17(1):65-82.

Park, G., Moon, E., Kim, D.W., & Lee, S.H. (2012). Individual differences in cardiac vagal tone are associated with differential neural responses to facial expressions at different spatial frequencies: an ERP and sLORETA study. Cogn Affect Behav Neurosci, Dec;12(4):777-93.

Park, S.M., Kim, H.J., Jang, S., et al. (2018). Depression is Closely Associated With Chronic Low Back Pain in Patients Over 50 Years of age: A Cross-sectional Study Using the Sixth Korea National Health and Nutrition Examination Survey (KNHANES VI-2). Spine (Phila Pa 1976). 2018 Feb 16. [Epub ahead of print].

Pelleymounter, M.A., Cullen, M.J., & Wellman, C.L. (1995). Characteristics of BDNF-induced weight loss. Exp Neurol, Feb;131(2):229-38.

Pereira, M.A., Kriska, A.M., Day, R.D., et al. (1998). A randomized walking trial in postmenopausal women: effects on physical activity and health 10 years later. Arch Intern Med, 158:1695-1701.

Pereira, A.C., Huddleston, D.E., Brickman, A.M., et al. (2007). An in vivo correlate of exercise-induced neurogenesis in the adult dentate gyrus. Proc Natl Acad Sci U S A., Mar 27; 104(13):5638-43.

Pinto Pereira, S.M., Ki, M., & Power, C. (2012). Sedentary behaviour and biomarkers for cardiovascular disease and diabetes in mid-life: the role of television-viewing and sitting at work. PLoS One, 7(2):e31132.

Petit, W.A., & Adamec, C. (2002). The encyclopedia of diabetes. New York: Facts on File.

Polyakova, M., Stuke, K., Schuemberg, K., et al. (2015). BDNF as a biomarker for successful treatment of mood disorders: a systematic & quantitative meta-analysis. J Affect Disord, Mar 15;174:432-40.

Pontzer, H. (2017). Economy and Endurance in Human Evolution. Curr Biol, Jun 19;27(12):R613-R621.

Price, K., Schartz, P., & Watson, A.H.D. (2014). The effect of standing and sitting postures on breathing in brass players. Springerplus, 3:210.

Pulsford, R.M., Blackwell, J., Hillsdon, M., & Kos, K. (2017). Intermittent walking, but not standing, improves postprandial insulin and glucose relative to sustained sitting: A randomised cross-over study in inactive middle-aged men. J Sci Med Sport, Mar;20(3):278-283.

Puterman, E., Lin, J., Blackburn, E., et al. (2010). The power of exercise: buffering the effect of chronic stress on telomere length. PLoS One, May 26;5(5):e10837.

Raczak, G., Pinna, G.D., La Rovere, M.T., et al. (2005). Cardiovagal response to acute mild exercise in young healthy subjects. Circ J, Aug;69(8):976-80.

Ranasinghe, P., Perera, Y.S., Lamabadusuriya, D.A., et al. (2011). Work related complaints of neck, shoulder and arm among computer office workers: a cross-sectional evaluation of prevalence and risk factors in a developing country. Environ Health, Aug 4;10:70.

Rapoport, J., Jacobs, P., Bell, N.R., & Klarenbach, S. (2004). Refining the measurement of the economic burden of chronic diseases in Canada. Chronic Dis Can, Winter;25(1):13-21.

Ratey, J. (2008). Spark: The Revolutionary New Science of Exercise and the Brain. Penguin Books.

Rawson, R.A., Chudzynski, J., Gonzales, R., et al. (2015). The Impact of

Exercise On Depression and Anxiety Symptoms Among Abstinent Methamphetamine-Dependent Individuals in A Residential Treatment Setting. J Subst Abuse Treat, Oct;57:36-40.

Reinehr, T. (2013). Type 2 diabetes mellitus in children and adolescents. World Journal of Diabetes, 4(6):270-281.

Renehan, A.G., Tyson, M., Egger, M., et al. (2008). Body-mass index and incidence of cancer: a systematic review and meta-analysis of prospective observational studies. Lancet, 371(9612):569-578.

Richards, M., Hardy, R., & Wadsworth, M.E. (2003). Does active leisure protect cognition? Evidence from a national birth cohort. Soc Sci Med, Feb; 56(4):785-92.

Rillamas-Sun, E., LaMonte, M.J., Evenson, K.R., et al. (2017). The Influence of Physical Activity and Sedentary Behavior on Living to Age 85 Years Without Disease and Disability in Older Women. J Gerontol A Biol Sci Med Sci, Nov 20. [Epub ahead of print].

Robertson, C.L., Ishibashi, K., Chudzynski, J., et al. (2016). Effect of Exercise Training on Striatal Dopamine D2/D3 Receptors in Methamphetamine Users during Behavioral Treatment. Neuropsychopharmacology, 41(6):1629–1636.

Rosecrance, J.C., Cook, T.M., & Zimmermann, C.L. (1996). Work-related musculoskeletal symptoms among construction workers in the pipe trades. Work, 7(1):13-20.

Rosenbaum, S., Sherrington, C., & Tiedemann, A. (2015). Exercise augmentation compared with usual care for post-traumatic stress disorder: a randomized controlled trial. Acta Psychiatr Scand, May;131(5):350-9.

Roussouly, P., & Pinheiro-Franco, J.L. (2011). Biomechanical analysis of the spino-pelvic organization and adaptation in pathology. Eur Spine J, Sep;20 Suppl 5:609-18.

Ruegsegger, G.N., & Booth, F.W. (2017). Running from Disease: Molecular Mechanisms Associating Dopamine and Leptin Signaling in the Brain with Physical Inactivity, Obesity, and Type 2 Diabetes. Front Endocrinol (Lausanne), May 23;8:109.

Ryan, T.M., & Shaw, C.N. (2015). Skeletal gracility in modern humans.

Proceedings of the National Academy of Sciences, Jan, 112 (2) 372-377.

Saeidifard, Farzane, et al. "Difference of Energy Expenditure While Standing versus Sitting: A Systematic Review and Meta-Analysis." (2017): A20539-A20539.

Sah, N., Peterson, B.D., Lubejko, S.T., et al. (2017). Running reorganizes the circuitry of one-week-old adult-born hippocampal neurons. Sci Rep, Sep 7;7(1):10903.

Saidj, M., Menai, M., Charreire, H., et al. (2015). Descriptive study of sedentary behaviours in 35,444 French working adults: cross-sectional findings from the ACTI-Cités study. BMC Public Health, Apr 14;15:379.

Sanfilippo, K.M., McTigue, K.M., Fidler, C.J., et al. (2014). Hypertension and obesity and the risk of kidney cancer in 2 large cohorts of US men and women. Hypertension, 63(5):934-41.

Saunders, T.J., Chaput, J.P., & Tremblay, M.S. (2014). Sedentary behaviour as an emerging risk factor for cardiometabolic diseases in children and youth. Can J Diabetes, Feb;38(1):53-61.

Scanlon, P.H. (2008). The English national screening programme for sight threatening diabetic retinopathy. Journal of Medical Screening, 15(1):1-4.

Schiltenwolf, M., Akbar, M., Neubauer, E., et al. (2017). The cognitive impact of chronic low back pain: Positive effect of multidisciplinary pain therapy. Scand J Pain, Oct;17:273-278.

Schmid, D., Leitzmann, M.F. (2014). Television Viewing and Time Spent Sedentary in Relation to Cancer Risk: A Meta-analysis. J Natl Cancer Inst, Jun 16;106(7).

Schoenfeld, T.J., & Cameron, H.A. (2015). Adult neurogenesis and mental illness. Neuropsychopharmacology, Jan;40(1):113-28.

Schoenfeld, T.J., Rada, P., Pieruzzini, P.R., et al. (2013). Physical exercise prevents stress-induced activation of granule neurons and enhances local inhibitory mechanisms in the dentate gyrus. J Neurosci, May 1;33(18):7770-7.

Schutte, N.M., Nederend, I., Hudziak, J.J., et al. (2017). Heritability of the affective response to exercise and its correlation to exercise behavior.

Psychol Sport Exerc, Jul;31:139-148.

Seip, R.L., & Semenkovich, C.F. (1998). Skeletal muscle lipoprotein lipase: molecular regulation and physiological effects in relation to exercise. Exerc Sport Sci Rev, 26:191-218.

Servant, D., Logier, R., Mouster, Y., & Goudemand, M. (2009). Heart rate variability. Applications in psychiatry. Encephale, Oct;35(5):423-8.

Setiawan, V.W., Yang, H.P., Pike, M.C., et al. (2013). Type I and II endometrial cancers: have they different risk factors? Journal of Clinical Oncology, 31(20):2607-2618.

Seuring, T., Archangelidi, O., Suhrcke, M. (2015). The economic costs of type 2 diabetes: A global systematic review. PharmacoEconomics, 33(8): 811–31.

Shahabi, L., Naliboff, B.D., Shapiro, D. (2016). Self-regulation evaluation of therapeutic yoga and walking for patients with irritable bowel syndrome: a pilot study. Psychol Health Med, 21(2):176-88.

Shan, J., Kushnir, A., Betzenhauser, M.J., et al. (2010). Phosphorylation of the ryanodine receptor mediates the cardiac fight or flight response in mice. J Clin Invest, Dec;120(12):4388-98.

Shevtsova, O., Tan, Y.F., Merkley, C.M., et al. (2017). Early-Age Running Enhances Activity of Adult-Born Dentate Granule Neurons Following Learning in Rats. eNeuro, Aug 16;4(4).

Shiri, R., Lallukka, T., Karppinen, J., & Viikari-Juntura, E. (2014). Obesity as a Risk Factor for Sciatica: A Meta-analysis. Am J Epidemiol, 179(8):929-937.

Shors, T., Anderson, L., Curlik, D.M., & Nokia, S. (2012). Use it or lose it: How neurogenesis keeps the brain fit for learning. Behavioural Brain Research, 227(2):450–458.

Shrestha, Nipun, et al. "Workplace interventions for reducing sitting at work." The Cochrane Library (2016).

Siddarth, P., Burggren, A.C., Eyre, H.A., et al. (2018). Sedentary behavior associated with reduced medial temporal lobe thickness in middle-aged and older adults. PLoS One, Apr 12;13(4):e0195549.

Simon, G.E., Von Korff, M., Saunders, K., et al. (2006). Association between obesity and psychiatric disorders in the US adult population. Archives of General Psychiatry, 63(7):824–830.

Smith, J.A., Fuino, R.L., Pesis-Katz, I., et al. (2017). Differences in opioid prescribing in low back pain patients with and without depression: a cross-sectional study of a national sample from the United States. Pain Rep, Jun 22;2(4):e606.

Smith, Peter, et al. "The relationship between occupational standing and sitting and incident heart disease over a 12-year period in Ontario, Canada." American journal of epidemiology 187.1 (2017): 27-33.

Sorlie, P.D., Kannel, W.B., & O'Connor, G. (1989). Mortality associated with respiratory function and symptoms in advanced age. The Framingham Study. Am Rev Respir Dis, Aug;140(2):379-84.

Stamatakis, E., Hamer, M., Dunstan, D.W. (2011). Screen-based entertainment time, all-cause mortality, and cardiovascular events: population-based study with ongoing mortality and hospital events follow-up. J Am Coll Cardiol, Jan 18;57(3):292-9.

Stewart, W.F., Ricci, J.A., Chee, E., et al. (2003). Lost productive time and cost due to common pain conditions in the US workforce. JAMA, Nov 12; 290(18):2443-54.

Stroke Association UK. (2016). State of the Nation - Stroke Statistics. Accessed February 15, 2016. Available: https://www.stroke.org.uk/sites/default/files/state_of_the_nation_2016_110116_0.pdf.

Stroth, S., Reinhardt, R.K., Thöne, J., et al. (2010). Impact of aerobic exercise training on cognitive functions and affect associated to the COMT polymorphism in young adults. Neurobiol Learn Mem, Oct; 94(3):364-72.

Stubbs, B., Vancampfort, D., Firth, J., et al. (2018). Relationship between sedentary behavior and depression: A mediation analysis of influential factors across the lifespan among 42,469 people in low- and middle-income countries. J Affect Disord. Mar 15;229:231-238.

Sturge-Apple, M.L., Suor, J.H., Davies, P.T., et al. (2016). Vagal Tone and Children's Delay of Gratification: Differential Sensitivity in Resource-Poor and Resource-Rich Environments. Psychol Sci, Jun;27(6):885-93.

Syväoja, H.J., Tammelin, T.H., Ahonen, T., et al. (2014). The associations of objectively measured physical activity and sedentary time with cognitive functions in school-aged children. PLoS One, 9(7):e103559.

Tanasescu, M., Leitzmann, M.F., Rimm, E.B., et al. (2002). Exercise type and intensity in relation to coronary heart disease in men. JAMA, Oct 23-30;288(16):1994-2000.

Thøgersen-Ntoumani, C., Loughren, E.A., Kinnafick, F.E., et al. (2015). Changes in work affect in response to lunchtime walking in previously physically inactive employees: A randomized trial. Scand J Med Sci Sports, Dec;25(6):778-87.

Thomas, E.L., Frost, G., Taylor-Robinson, S.D., & Bell, J.D. (2012). Excess body fat in obese and normal-weight subjects. Nutr Res Rev, Jun;25(1):150-61.

Toro, A.L., Costantino, N.S., Shriver, C.D., et al. (2016). Effect of obesity on molecular characteristics of invasive breast tumors: gene expression analysis in a large cohort of female patients. BMC Obesity, 3, 22.

Trejo, J.L., Carro, E., Torres-Aleman, I. (2001). Circulating insulin-like growth factor I mediates exercise-induced increases in the number of new neurons in the adult hippocampus. J Neurosci, Mar 1;21(5):1628-34.

Tsai, S.F., Ku, N.W., Wang, T.F., et al. (2018). Long-Term Moderate Exercise Rescues Age-Related Decline in Hippocampal Neuronal Complexity and Memory. Gerontology, May 7:1-11.

Van der Ploeg, Hidde P., et al. "Sitting time and all-cause mortality risk in 222 497 Australian adults." Archives of internal medicine 172.6 (2012): 494-500.

Vasiliadis, H.M., & Bélanger, M.F. (2018). The prospective and concurrent effect of exercise on health related quality of life in older adults over a 3 year period. Health Qual Life Outcomes, Jan 16;16(1):15.

Wallin, A., & Larsson, S.C. (2011). Body mass index and risk of multiple myeloma: a meta-analysis of prospective studies. European Journal of Cancer, 47(11):1606-1615.

Wallmann-Sperlich, Birgit, et al. "Who uses height-adjustable desks?-Sociodemographic, health-related, and psycho-social variables of regular users." International Journal of Behavioral Nutrition and Physical Activity 14.1 (2017): 26.

Wang, F., & Xu, Y. (2014). Body mass index and risk of renal cell cancer: a dose-response meta-analysis of published cohort studies. International Journal of Cancer, 135(7):1673-86.

Warren, T.Y., Barry, V., Hooker, S.P., et al. (2010). Sedentary behaviors increase risk of cardiovascular disease mortality in men. Med Sci Sports Exerc, May;42(5):879-85.

Warrener, A.G. (2017). Hominin Hip Biomechanics: Changing Perspectives. Anat Rec (Hoboken), May;300(5):932-945.

Waters, Thomas R., and Robert B. Dick. "Evidence of health risks associated with prolonged standing at work and intervention effectiveness." Rehabilitation Nursing 40.3 (2015): 148-165.

Webber, J.T., & Raichlen, D.A. (2016). The role of plantigrady and heel-strike in the mechanics and energetics of human walking with implications for the evolution of the human foot. J Exp Biol, Dec 1;219(Pt 23):3729-3737.

WebMD. (2011). Is sitting too long a major cancer risk? Published Nov 3, 2011. Accessed April 2018. Available: https://www.webmd.com/cancer/news/20111103/is-sitting-too-long-a-major-cancer-risk#1.

Wens, I., Keytsman, C., Deckx, N., et al. (2016). Brain derived neurotrophic factor in multiple sclerosis: effect of 24 weeks endurance and resistance training. Eur J Neurol, Jun;23(6):1028-35.

Werneck, A.O., Cyrino, E.S., Collings, P.J., et al. (2018). TV Viewing in 60,202 Adults From the National Brazilian Health Survey: Prevalence, Correlates, and Associations With Chronic Diseases. J Phys Act Health, Mar 15:1-6.

Wilmot, E.G., Edwardson, C.L., Achana, F.A. et al. (2012). Sedentary time in adults and the association with diabetes, cardiovascular disease and death: systematic review and meta-analysis. Diabetologia, Nov, 55(11):2895–2905.

Winter, B., Breitenstein, C., Mooren, F.C., et al. (2007). High impact running improves learning. Neurobiol Learn Mem, May;87(4):597-609.

Wirth, B., Amstalden, M., Perk, M., et al. (2014). Respiratory dysfunction in patients with chronic neck pain - influence of thoracic spine and chest mobility. Man Ther, Oct;19(5):440-4.

Wirth, B., Ferreira, T.D., Mittelholzer, M., et al. (2016). Respiratory muscle endurance training reduces chronic neck pain: A pilot study. J Back Musculoskelet Rehabil, Nov 21;29(4):825-834.

Wong, E., Backholer, K., Gearon, E., et al. (2013). Diabetes and risk of physical disability in adults: a systematic review and meta-analysis. Lancet Diabetes Endocrinology, 1:(2)106–114.

World Cancer Research Fund International/American Institute for Cancer Research. (2015). Continuous Update Project Report: Diet, Nutrition, Physical Activity and Gallbladder Cancer. Accessed March 2018. Available at http://www.wcrf.org/sites/default/files/Gallbladder-Cancer-2015-Report.pdf.

World Health Organization. (2016). Global Report on Diabetes. Accessed March 2018. Available: http://apps.who.int/iris/bitstream/10665/204871/1/9789241565257_eng.pdf.

World Heath Organization. (2017). Top 10 Causes of Death. 2017. Accessed March 2018. Available: http://www.who.int/mediacentre/factsheets/fs310/en/.

World Health Organization (2003). Nutrition: Controlling the global obesity epidemic. Press release, published 23 April 2003. Accessed March 2018. Available: http://www.who.int/nutrition/topics/obesity/en/.

Wu, C., Garamszegi, S.P., Xie, X., & Mash, D.C. (2017). Altered Dopamine Synaptic Markers in Postmortem Brain of Obese Subjects. Front Hum Neurosci, Aug 3;11:386.

Xie, Y., Szeto, G., & Dai, J. (2017). Prevalence and risk factors associated with musculoskeletal complaints among users of mobile handheld devices: A systematic review. Appl Ergon, Mar;59(Pt A):132-142.

Yaffe, K., Fiocco, A.J., Lindquist, K., et al. (2009). Predictors of maintaining cognitive function in older adults: the Health ABC study. Neurology, Jun 9; 72(23):2029-35.

Younossi, Z.M., & Henry, L. (2015). Economic and quality-of-life implications of non-alcoholic fatty liver disease. PharmacoEconomics, 33:1245–1253.

YouTube. What is the second biggest preventable cause of cancer after smoking? Uploaded February 23, 2018. Accessed April 22, 2018. Available: https://www.youtube.com/watch?v=6v2mDFTo6ao&feature=youtu.be.

Zang, J., Liu, Y., Li, W., et al. (2017). Voluntary exercise increases adult hippocampal neurogenesis by increasing GSK-3ß activity in mice. Neuroscience, Jun 23;354:122-135.

Zeki, A.l., Hazzouri, A., Caunca, M.R., et al. (2018). Greater depressive symptoms, cognition, and markers of brain aging: Northern Manhattan Study. Neurology, May 9. pii: 10.1212/WNL.0000000000005639. [Epub ahead of print].

ABOUT THE AUTHOR

Eric Soehngen, MD, PhD, FAWM is a board certified physician, researcher and company owner. Medically, he is dedicated to researching the health effects of lack of exercise in the workplace. He is considered the founder and inventor of the "work and walk" concept. In 2017, together with co-founder Frank Ackermann, he launched the company WALKOLUTION - the world's first medical research-based active workplace solution that enables users to keep moving naturally while they work.

Together with renowned experts in the fields of ergonomics, evolutionary biology and the life sciences, he develops concepts for medical and neurocognitive optimized workplaces. He believes that movement is a fundamental right of man and that it needs to be recognized as a medical necessity. As a mountaineer and trail runner, he finds his personal dose of exercise in the Alps of his Bavarian home.

Made in United States
Orlando, FL
10 June 2022

18687274R00085